Beyond the Mask: Autism in Africa

Chopra

Table of Contents

Chapter One - Introduction

1.1. Introduction

This chapter begins by stating the research problem and providing a rationale for conducting the research. Thereafter, the research problem has been formulated, key concepts clarified, and ethical considerations of the study discussed.

1.2. Statement of the Problem

Autism Spectrum Disorder (ASD) only emerged as a point of discussion within a global context in recent decades (Donvan & Zucker, 2016). ASD is a developmental disorder that has increased in prevalence (Centers for Disease Control and Prevention, 2014a). Due to the rapidity in which the prevalence of ASD has increased, ASD has now become viewed as an epidemic (Eyal, Hart, Onculer, Oren & Rossi, 2010). Reasons for this increase have included increased clarity on diagnostic criteria, an increase in ASD awareness, and an increase of professionals qualified to diagnose ASD (Eyal et al., 2010). However, the most likely reason for the increase in prevalence is due to the broad diagnostic boundaries of ASD, which has resulted in many children who struggle socially being misdiagnosed with ASD (Eyal et al., 2010).

A global study estimated that one in 132 people live with ASD (Baxter, Brugha, Erskine, Scheurer, Vos & Scott, 2015). However, research conducted by the Centers for Disease Control and Prevention (2018) found that up to one in 59 children in the United States of America (USA) live with ASD, with a higher prevalence found in boys than girls. One possible reason for the variance between the prevalence found globally and the prevalence found within the USA is the different strategies used to identify those living with ASD (Baxter et al., 2015). Global studies have largely used registry data to work out prevalence, while other studies have used more comprehensive means (Baxter et al., 2015). Unfortunately, there has not seemed to be an indication of the prevalence of ASD within an African or South African context. The lack of information on prevalence within South Africa has been noted in studies by Chambers et al. (2016) and Van Biljion, Kritzinger and Geertsema (2015). A scarcity of literature also exists with regard to the history of ASD and mental health care within Africa and South Africa.

According to Breen, Swartz, Flisher, Joska, Corrigall, Plaatjies and McDonald (2007), the burden of caring for children living with disabilities within South Africa has fallen onto the family system. This has left parents to navigate the demands of caring for their children living with mental health disorders, such as ASD. However, there has seemed to be a lack of knowledge and a high level of stigmatisation linked to ASD, which has led to little support for parents in caring for these children (Corcoran, Berry & Hill, 2015; DePape & Lindsay, 2015; Selman, Fox, Aabe, Turner, Rai & Redwood, 2017). In previous studies, diagnosis has usually occurred during early childhood, and parents have been faced with having to understand ASD, decide on how to proceed with the child's care, and deal with ASD-related challenges (Silverman, 2012; DePape & Lindsay, 2015). Due to the high burden of care for parents with children living with ASD, and the lack of support from others, it could be concluded that caring for a child living with ASD within South Africa could have a unique set of stressors, leading to the need for specific coping strategies (Breen et al., 2007).

There has been a paucity of literature that has explored the general experiences of parents of children living with ASD within South Africa (Monare, 2015), making it difficult for health care professionals (HCPs) to understand their experiences, and how to support them as a result. HCPs, in this context, are those health care professionals who come into contact with, or work with, children living with ASD. This includes those registered with both the Health Professions Council of South Africa (HCPSA) and the South African Council for Social Service Professions (SACSSP), the latter includes Social Workers. More specifically, there is a lack of research on the stressors and resulting coping mechanisms of parents with children living with ASD within South Africa. Therefore, this study explored the experiences of parents who care for children living with ASD within South Africa, and focussed on the specific stressors experienced, coping mechanisms employed, and support mechanisms needed.

1.3. Rationale of the Research

The gap in research on the experiences of parents caring for a child living with ASD (Monare, 2015) exists alongside the shift of care falling more onto these parents (Breen et al., 2007). This necessitates more research in this area, since there is a lack of knowledge and a simultaneous increase in need. Therefore, this study answers Monare's (2015) call to further research being conducted on the experiences and challenges of parents raising children living with ASD within a South African context.

There are numerous practical benefits of this research. One benefit is that this study could provide HCPs and other professionals working within the ASD field with an increased understanding of parents' actual experiences, including their stressors, coping mechanisms, and need for support. This increase in understanding would assist HCPs and other professionals working within the ASD field to provide more appropriate services to suit the specific needs of these parents. Specifically for Social Workers, this would also indicate where the gaps exist in working with the child and their family to understand what they are facing and to appropriately provide support to them. Aside from HCPs and other professionals, this study could increase the general awareness of the realities of caring for a child living with ASD, so as to decrease stigmatisation within communities and increase appropriate support for parents.

This study could also benefit other parents caring for a child living with ASD, as it may normalise the challenges that they experience. This aligns with Behane's (2016) finding that one of the coping mechanisms that parents have utilised in caring for their children is support from others who have faced similar circumstances. This study also provides education to parents caring for a child living with ASD so that they are able to better cope with the stressors that they experience, as well as gives them ideas as to how to cope and gain more support. This is essential, as Tadesse (2014) found that, after a child has been diagnosed as living with ASD, parents are often ill-equipped or uneducated on how to cope with their child's diagnosis.

1.4. Research Topic
The research topic for this study is: An exploration into the stressors and coping strategies of parents caring for children living with ASD.

1.5. Main Research Questions
The main research questions for this study are:
    1.5.1. What stressors are faced by parents of children living with ASD?
    1.5.2. What coping strategies do parents use in caring for children living with ASD?
    1.5.3. What support mechanisms do parents of children living with ASD need to cope effectively?

1.6. Research Objectives

The research objectives for this study are:

1.6.1. To explore the stressors faced by parents of children living with ASD.

1.6.2. To explore the coping strategies that parents use in caring for children living with ASD.

1.6.3. To determine what support mechanisms parents of children living with ASD need to cope effectively.

1.7. Concept Clarification

Autism Spectrum Disorder (ASD): ASD is a neurodevelopmental disorder that can be identified by a deficiency in social communication and interactions (American Psychiatric Association, 2013). ASD is usually diagnosed between the ages of 2 and 4 years old (Centers for Disease Control and Prevention, 2014b; Crane, Chester, Goddard, Henry & Hill, 2015). Its symptoms include communication difficulties, delayed speech, and sensory perception difficulties (Centers for Disease Control and Prevention, 2014b). ASD usually includes the presence of repetitive behaviours, such as repetitively lining up objects (Centers for Disease Control and Prevention, 2014b).

Child: A child is a person under the age of 18 years old (Children's Act, No. 38 of 2005, 2006). In this study it referred to a child living with ASD, unless otherwise specified.

Health Care Professional (HCP): A HCP is a person who provides and promotes health care to others (World Health Organisation, 2020). In this study, this includes those registered with both the HPCSA and the SACSSP within South Africa. Social Workers are HCPs registered with the SACSSP.

Parent: A parent is either biological or adoptive, and has full legal responsibilities and rights to the child (Children's Act, No. 38 of 2005, 2006). In this study, it referred to the biological or adoptive primary caregivers of a child living with ASD, unless otherwise specified.

Stressor: A stressor is an event that could lead, or has led, to harm or loss, or that presents a challenge (Folkman & Lazarus, 1980). In this study, it specifically referred to the stressors experienced by parents of children living with ASD.

Coping strategies: Coping strategies are ways in which people behave and think to deal with the threat of a stressful situation (Folkman & Lazarus, 1980). In this study, it specifically referred to coping strategies employed by parents of children living with ASD.

Support mechanism: A support mechanism is an external protective factor, which results in resiliency and increases a person's ability to cope when faced with difficulties (Greene, Galambos & Lee, 2004). In this study, it specifically referred to the support mechanisms needed or utilised by parents of children living with ASD.

1.8. Ethical Considerations

Ethical considerations are of utmost importance, as research should be accurate and never be done at the expense of human beings (De Vos, Strydom & Delport, 2011). The ethical considerations pertinent to this study are outlined below.

1.8.1. Informed consent

To enable respondents to make an informed decision about consenting to being part of a study, respondents need to be given accurate information and all necessary details that pertain to the study (De Vos et al., 2011). One way of doing this is to give respondents a consent form (Appendix A) that includes all necessary information that can enable them to make an informed decision as to whether or not to take part (De Vos et al., 2011). Taking this into consideration, this study utilised a consent form to outline the aim of the research, what would be done with information collected, the use of a digital recording device, and the nature of privacy, confidentiality and anonymity that would be maintained throughout. A copy of the consent form was sent to respondents via email prior to being interviewed so that they could familiarise themselves with its content, and ask any questions they had.

De Vos et al. (2011) highlighted the need for the researcher to ensure that respondents have a clear understanding of the consent form before consenting to be part of a study. In line with this, at the outset of each interview, the researcher in this study ensured that respondents had read the consent form and answered any questions respondents had before they signed consent to participate. If respondents were satisfied with the consent form and signed it, then the interview went ahead. For those who were interviewed telephonically, the consent form was signed remotely before the interview took place, and was scanned and emailed back to the researcher before the interview. In this study all respondents consented.

1.8.2. Voluntary participation

Since respondents are sharing their personal information for the purposes of research, their consent must be completely voluntary and void of incentive or coercion (De Vos et al., 2011). The researcher must therefore ensure that respondents are involved of their own free will and are enabled to withdraw at any stage during the research process (De Vos et al., 2011). To cater for this, the consent form in this study highlighted that respondents' involvement was voluntary, that they could change their minds at any stage in the process, and that no compensation for participation would be given. Furthermore, the researcher maintained a neutral tone in approaching potential participants and reiterated the voluntary nature of this study so that respondents did not feel coerced into participating.

1.8.3. Avoidance of harm to respondents

Any physical and emotional harm to respondents needs to be avoided during research (De Vos et al., 2011). There was no risk of physical harm to respondents within this study. However, the avoidance of emotional harm was especially important as the topic of this study was of a personal nature. The researcher avoided emotional harm by only asking questions relevant to the study, and more emotive questions were asked later in the interview once rapport was built. If a respondent became emotional while being interviewed, the interviewer paused and asked the respondent if they would like to continue. If the respondent had not wanted to continued, the researcher would have contained the respondent and ended the interview. The respondent would have been referred if necessary. If the respondent wanted to continue, the researcher diverted the line of questioning, as suggested by De Vos et al. (2011). In this study, only one respondent became noticeably emotional during the interview. However, the respondent chose to continue and a referral was recommended for possible unprocessed grief.

1.8.4. Debriefing of respondents

Debriefing consists of working through respondents' experiences of, and feelings towards, their interview with the researcher (De Vos et al., 2011). Debriefing after the interview can bring closure to the interview process and is another way in which harm can be avoided

(De Vos et al., 2011). In this study, after each interview, respondents were debriefed to explore how they experienced the interview to minimise any potential emotional harm. Respondents asked any questions they had and, if necessary, clarity was provided on the research to avoid any misperceptions that might have occurred. When necessary, options for referral were discussed.

1.8.5. Privacy, anonymity and confidentiality of respondents

1.8.5.1. Privacy

Privacy refers to the right of respondents to determine what they reveal and who they reveal it to (De Vos et al., 2011). The privacy of respondents is of utmost importance and needs to be maintained as much as possible (De Vos et al., 2011). In this study, the researcher endeavoured to maintain respondents' privacy, especially due to the personal nature of the interviews. The researcher ensured that face-to-face interviews took place in a private setting, which was usually in respondents' homes.

Before interviewing respondents telephonically, Mealer and Jones (2014) highlighted the importance of making respondents aware that they need to be interviewed in a private space where they feel comfortable and will not be disturbed. In this study, when an interview took place over Skype, the researcher ensured that she, herself, was in a private space. Before the interview was scheduled, the researcher also asked these respondents to find a private space where they would feel comfortable. The researcher explained to these respondents that a 'private space' referred to a place where the interview could not be overheard or disturbed by others.

1.8.5.2. Anonymity

Complete anonymity means that the identity of respondents is not known to anyone, including the researcher, at any time during the research process (De Vos et al., 2011). As this study utilised a qualitative research design, complete anonymity could not be ensured. Respondents were made aware that their identities would only be known to the researcher.

The purpose of anonymity is to protect the identity of the individual from being linked to the findings of the study (De Vos et al., 2011). As complete anonymity was not possible in this study, the researcher attempted to create privacy in other ways. Privacy was ensured by emailing respondents on their private email addresses so that only they had access to the particulars of the interview, and interviews were conducted in private settings. According to Sadler, Lee, Lim and Fullerton (2010), snowball sampling inherently risks the privacy and anonymity of respondents, as personal information is disclosed as one respondent asks another person if they would like to participate in the study. The researcher therefore needs to do their best in keeping the privacy and anonymity of respondents obtained when utilising this sampling method (Sadler et al., 2010). In an attempt to adhere to Sadlers et al.'s (2010) sentiments, the researcher ensured there was no information in the research report that could allow others to deduce the identity of other respondents, including those who they might have recommended as respondents for the study.

1.8.5.3. Confidentiality

Confidentiality implies that, at all times, only a select number of people, usually consisting of the researcher and their staff, know respondents' identities (De Vos et al., 2011). In this study, the researcher was the only person who knew the identity of respondents. The researcher ensured confidentiality by locking the recording device away when not in use, password protecting digital identifying data, and ensuring that the report did not include identifying particulars. Interviews were transcribed by the researcher and any identifying information was omitted, further ensuring that no one beside the researcher was able to identify respondents.

1.8.6. Competency and experience of the researcher

The researcher has to be competent due to prior knowledge and experience, as well as remain objective and ensure referencing is correct (De Vos et al., 2011). In this study, the researcher had previous experience from the completion of a Bachelor of Social Work, which had included conducting a research project. The masters degree, to which this study forms a part, also included various expert-level interviewing skills, which were used within this study. According to De Vos et al. (2011), one way of ensuring that the researcher remains objective is to discuss their work with colleagues. Within this study, a university supervisor guided the researcher during the research process, and held the researcher accountable, including ensuring the researcher's objectivity. Correct referencing within a study is important as it allows others to access the original source that is being drawn from (De Vos et al., 2011). The researcher ensured referencing was done correctly by referring to a reference guide, and asked her supervisor if additional questions arose.

1.9. Conclusion

This chapter outlined the statement of the problem and rationale of the research. It then presented the research topic, main research questions and objectives, followed by concept clarification and the ethical considerations of the study.

Chapter Two - Literature Review

2.1. Introduction

This chapter presents the literature reviewed and the theoretical framework underpinning this study. The policy and legislation pertaining to this study is also covered.

2.2. Review of the Literature

2.2.1. ASD diagnosis

The causes of ASD are unclear (Eyal et al., 2010). ASD was initially thought to be caused by a mother's coldness towards her child, but this has since been refuted (Donvan and Zucker, 2016). Currently, a reason for the lack of clarity with regards to the causes of ASD could be due to the use of ASD as a catchall for numerous social challenges children experience (McGeer, 2010). This may have led to a wide range of profiles of those diagnosed with ASD (McGeer, 2010). It has also been argued that ASD could be a part of neurodiversity, whereby it is a natural variation within one's neurological makeup (Donvan & Zucker, 2016). Whilst some agree with the previous two explanations, it has been agreed that ASD is linked to genetic or biological factors (McGeer, 2010).

The symptoms of ASD exist on a spectrum (McGeer, 2010). According to Eyal et al. (2010), because ASD exists on a spectrum, many different intervention options are needed. As ASD varies from person-to-person, the blend of interventions used is therefore unique (National Institute of Mental Health USA, 2018). However, one of the concerns with regard to the unique blend of interventions each child could benefit from, is that previous studies have found that many parents caring for children living with ASD struggle to access appropriate intervention strategies due a myriad of reasons (Chirwa, 2012; Corcoran, Berry & Hill, 2015; DePape & Lindsay, 2015; Berhane, 2016).

Due to the lack of consensus in the field with regard to the causes of ASD (Eyal et al., 2010) and ASD having been used as a catchall diagnosis (McGeer, 2010), it can be assumed that the process of ascertaining a diagnosis of ASD could be a difficult experience for caregivers of children living with ASD.

2.2.2. Parents' experiences of the diagnostic process

Reaching an ASD diagnosis is a difficult process that parents need to navigate (Crane et al., 2015). It has been found to cause high levels of stress in parents, especially due to the usual delay in receiving an official diagnosis (DePape & Lindsay, 2015). Reasons for late diagnosis include having received an initial misdiagnosis and having to rule out other possible diagnoses (DePape & Lindsay, 2015). It has also been found that parents experience many negative emotions during the diagnostic process, including feelings of guilt, anxiety, and loss (Crane et al., 2015; Berhane, 2016; Burrell, Ives & Unwin, 2017; Chao et al., 2017). Loss has been found to centre around the loss of parents' future dreams and expectations for their children (Chao et al., 2017).

Although the diagnostic process was found to lead to many negative emotions, positive emotions have been found too (Tadesse, 2014; Corcoran, Berry & Hill, 2015; Berhane, 2016). Positive emotions were due to the fact that many parents experienced relief, as they finally had clarity and a diagnosis for their child's behaviours (DePape & Lindsay, 2015). Furthermore, receiving the diagnosis has resulted in increased feelings of empowerment (Chao et al., 2017). Consequently, it can be concluded that the diagnostic process results in a myriad of emotions for parents. One of the ways in which parents sought to gain control post-diagnosis, was by educating themselves on ASD (Burrel, Ives & Unwin, 2017).

2.2.2.1. Parents' efforts to increase their understanding of ASD

Many parents made an effort to increase their understanding of ASD as a form of coping after receiving their child's diagnosis (Kuhaneck et al., 2010; Marshall & Long, 2010; Berhane, 2016; Burrell, Ives & Unwin, 2017; Selman et al., 2017). Self-education was therefore found to be paramount to being able to cope with their child's needs (Kuhaneck et al., 2010). Some did this through their interactions with various HCPs (Selman et al., 2017), whilst others spoke to fellow parents who also had children living with ASD (Berhane, 2016). An increase in knowledge may have also enabled parents to more readily accept their child's diagnosis (Berhane, 2016). Self-education was also said to possibly decrease parents' feelings of powerlessness, and in this way could have contributed to an increased ability to cope (Marshall & Long, 2010).

2.2.2.2. Parents' acceptance of their child's ASD diagnosis

The need for parents to come to a place of acceptance of their child's ASD diagnosis was found to be a very important step in the journey of caring for their child (DePape & Lindsay, 2015; Burrell, Ives & Unwin, 2017). Making ASD a normal part of family life was one of the ways in which acceptance could be found (DePape & Lindsay, 2015). Additionally, reframing ASD and what it meant for themselves was another way in which parents were able to come to a place of acceptance (Tadesse, 2014; Selman et al., 2017). However, since ASD could lead to judgement and being excluded by others, reaching acceptance of ASD was found to be especially difficult for parents (Chirwa, 2012; Selman et al., 2017). Nevertheless, a study on a Somalian community living in the United Kingdom, found that acceptance enabled parents to cope better with stigmatisation (Selman et al., 2017). Furthermore, Burrell, Ives and Unwin (2017) found that acceptance led to a decrease in parents' internalisation of others' responses to their child's diagnosis.

2.2.3. Challenges experienced by parents caring for children living with ASD

Parents experience various challenges in caring for children living with ASD. These challenges include dealing with their children's difficult behaviours, stigmatisation, the emotional impact of ASD on parents, financial strain, finding appropriate schooling for their children, and experiencing anxiety regarding their children's futures.

2.2.3.1. Difficult behaviours

Many of the behaviours included in the definition of ASD have been found to be particularly difficult for parents to deal with (Valicenti-McDermott, Lawson, Hottinger, Seijo, Schechtman, Shulman & Shinnar, 2015; Berhane, 2016). Examples of these behaviours include needing to deal with their children's high levels of irritability (Valicenti-McDermott et al.) and their socially inappropriate behaviours when in public (Berhane, 2016). Multiple studies found that attempting to manage these difficult, ASD-related behaviours was related to high stress levels in parents (Shawler & Sullivan, 2015; Valicenti-McDermott et al., 2015; Berhane, 2016). Apart from stress, other negative emotions experienced by parents in this regard have included: embarrassment when difficult behaviours have occurred in public, frustration, anger, and guilt (Burrell, Ives & Unwin, 2017).

2.2.3.2. Stigmatisation experienced by parents

Stigmatisation is a key challenge faced by many parents caring for a child living with ASD (Selman et al., 2017). Despite an increase in ASD awareness (Donvan & Zucker, 2016), a lack of understanding of ASD is still the primary reason for stigmatisation (Selman et al., 2017). On the African continent, certain communities in Ethiopia had still not heard of ASD when a study was conducted by Tadesse (2014), and within a Somalian community there was no word in their language that could be used to refer to ASD (Selman et al., 2017). In South Africa, a study on mothers found that stigmatisation had a negative impact on their lives (Van der Merwe, 2012). This stigma was found to mainly result from their child's difficult behaviours that often occurred without other people being able to tell that their child was living with ASD and judging them as a result.

Parents were found to respond to stigmatisation in a variety of different ways. Many avoided going out to public places due to feelings of embarrassment and frustration, resulting in isolation (Corcoran, Berry & Hill, 2015). While some parents ignored perceived stigmatisation from others, other parents confronted it (DePape & Lindsay, 2015). Many parents also felt judged as a result of feeling stigmatised (DePape & Lindsay, 2015; Selman et al., 2017). Feelings of judgement were especially found to come from HCPs, extended family members, and other parents who did not have children living with ASD (DePape & Lindsay, 2015; Selman et al., 2017).

2.2.3.3. The emotional impact of ASD on parents

Many studies found that having a child living with ASD could be emotionally taxing and could lead to high levels of negative emotion (Smith, Hong, Seltzer, Greenberg, Almeida & Bishop, 2010; Corcoran, Berry & Hill, 2015; Marciano, Drasgow & Carlson, 2015). One example is the high levels of stress that were found in many parents, especially when children were unable to verbally communicate (Marciano, Drasgow & Carlson, 2015). This stress was found to be due to the child not being able to express their needs (Tadesse, 2014). It was also found that high stress levels could lead to a decrease in resilience and the ability to cope (Kavaliotis, 2017). As a result, parents were found to be more susceptible to depression, anxiety, and exhaustion (Tadesse, 2014). In a study by Seltzer, Greenberg, Hong, Smith, Almeida, Coe and Stawski (2010), the cortisol levels of mothers who cared for children with ASD was found to be comparable to cortisol levels in combat soldiers, people who survived the Holocaust, and those who suffered from post-traumatic stress disorder. However, when looking at the high levels of stress in parents, Whitmore (2016) warned that one cannot separate different types of stressors from one's overall level of stress, making it difficult to pinpoint exactly what portion of parents' stress is due to caring for a child living with ASD.

2.2.3.4. Financial strain on parents

In many studies it was found that parents experienced financial strain due to their child's diagnosis (Centers for Disease Control and Prevention, 2014a; Tadesse, 2014; Kavaliotis, 2017). An example of a reason for financial strain is he need to provide specialised childcare and interventions for their child (Tadesse, 2014). Reasons for financial strain also included having a single income in the home (Tadesse, 2014; Berhane, 2016), high treatment costs (Hartley et al., 2016; Kavaliotis, 2017), special diets, finding appropriate schooling, and high transport costs to get to these schools (Tadesse, 2014).

As a result of financial strain, some parents within South Africa have been given access to government grants for their children (Burrell, Ives & Unwin, 2017). Within South Africa there are two grants available to children. The first is the child support grant, which is available to a primary caregiver of any South African child who falls within the parameters of the means test, is given regardless of diagnosis, and amounted to R420 per month, per child, in October 2019 (Mboweni, 2019). The second is the care dependency grant, which provides for any South African child who has a severe disability, falls within the means test, and needs full-time special care, which amounted to R1 780 per month, per child, in 2019 (Mboweni, 2019). Both of the above grant amounts are subject to a slight annual increase (Mboweni, 2019). While these grants may help parents who fall within the means test, the requirements to gain access would exclude many parents who do not meet this test, yet who are still facing financial strain. Additionally, the Rand value of these grants may not decrease financial strain, as they are very low considering the cost of living in South Africa (Numbeo, 2017).

2.2.3.5. The challenge to find appropriate schooling for their children

Parents have the challenge of finding appropriate, specialised and affordable schooling for their children, especially as most cost-effective, mainstream schooling is often unable to cater to their children (Rubenstein, Schelling, Wilczynski & Hooks, 2015; Johansson, 2016; Burrell, Ives & Unwin, 2017). Many studies found that parents needed to advocate in order to gain acceptance for their child into the school of their choice, as well as to have their child's educational needs met (Rubenstein et al., 2015; Johansson, 2016; Burrell, Ives & Unwin, 2017). As a result of this need to advocate, finding appropriate schooling for one's child was found to lead to an increase in stress and anxiety for parents (Rubenstein et al., 2015). Some parents have also been found to resort to homeschooling their children to deal with this challenge (Hurlbutt, 2011; Olatunji, 2014). While parents were found to experience anxiety regarding finding appropriate schooling for their children, they were also found to experience anxiety regarding their children's futures (Burrell, Ives & Unwin, 2017).

2.2.3.6. Parents' anxieties regarding their children's futures

Parents were found to experience multiple anxieties with regards to their children's futures (Burrell, Ives & Unwin, 2017). One of their greatest anxieties was who would look after their child if something were to happen to them as the parent (Tadesse, 2014; Berhane, 2016). Parents also expressed concern that their child would be less accepted as they got older and their symptoms became more obvious in contrast to other adolescents and adults (Marciano, Drasgow & Carlson, 2015). Concern also centred around difficulties their child might experience in finding employment (DePape & Lindsay, 2015; Burrell, Ives & Unwin, 2017). Additionally, parents had to deal with the loss of future dreams that they had for their child before their child was diagnosed as living with ASD (Corcoran, Berry & Hill, 2015; Crane et al., 2015; DePape & Lindsay, 2015).

2.2.4. Coping mechanisms and support needed by parents of children living with ASD

Aside from some of the coping mechanisms that have already been discussed, others have included gaining support from others, educating others on ASD, learning to manage their children's difficult behaviours, and personal growth.

2.2.4.1. Gaining support from others

Attaining support from others seems to be one of the main ways in which parents attempt to cope with caring for a child living with ASD (Corcoran, Berry & Hill, 2015). Feeling supported socially had been found to lead to a decrease in stress and an increase in parents' abilities to adjust (Siman-Tov & Kaniel, 2011). Due to stigmatisation and a lack of ASD-related knowledge within communities, many parents struggled to find adequate support to cope effectively (Corcoran, Berry & Hill, 2015; Berhane, 2016; Burrell, Ives & Unwin, 2017).

Some studies found that parents gained informal means of support through other parents who also had children living with ASD (Berhane, 2016; Burrell, Ives & Unwin, 2017). This was believed to have been a result of being able to be honest with one another about their struggles (Burrell, Ives & Unwin, 2017). This support was found to normalise what parents were going through, and gave them hope for the future (Berhane, 2016). It has been suggested that HCPs refer parents to support groups, especially if parents are susceptible to high levels of stress, depression, and anxiety (Crane et al., 2015). However, Burrell, Ives and Unwin (2017) found that some fathers found support groups to be too impersonal, and merely educational.

Corcoran, Berry and Hill's (2015) research found that spousal support was the biggest form of support that parents reported receiving. This was confirmed in another study, where many parents felt supported by their spouses through their challenge of caring for their child (Hartley, DaWalt & Schultz, 2017). Hall and Graff (2010) found that extended family members also provided support for parents. However, in a study conducted by Blanche et al. (2015), it was found that although extended family members were a form of support for parents, they were often slow and resistant to accepting the child's diagnosis of ASD. Blanche et al. (2015) also found that the extended familial support that mothers received was mostly from other female family members.

Ammari, Morris and Schoenebeck (2014) found that parents of children living with disabilities used Facebook most often as their social media platform of choice, with the predominant purpose of seeking social support. One of the reasons for seeking support through this medium was the perception that there was less judgement from others, making it a safer space than alternate forms (Ammari, Morris & Schoenebeck, 2014).

2.2.4.2. Educating others on ASD
The concept of educating others on ASD as a form of coping is one that has been found in various studies (Kuhaneck et al., 2010; Marshall & Long, 2010; Neely-Barnes, Hall, Roberts & Graff, 2011; Lutz, Patterson & Klein, 2012). According to Marshall and Long (2010), educating others has been found to be utilized as a coping strategy against the

perceived judgement from, and ignorance, of others. It has also been found to help parents cope with others' negative comments about their child's ASD-related behaviours (Neely-Barnes et al., 2011). Parents have especially spent time educating their family members (Kuhaneck et al., 2010; Lutz, Patterson & Klein, 2012), and have attempted to educate those within their communities (Kuhaneck et al., 2010; Lutz, Patterson & Klein, 2012). However, Neely-Barnes et al. (2011) also found that while many parents attempted to educate others, there were still some who avoided addressing ASD publically for fear of others' reactions. A recommendation that Kavaliotis (2017) made was for HCPs to be the ones to increase awareness of the realities of families living with ASD within communities, so as to increase social support for parents.

2.2.4.3. Learning to manage their children's challenging behaviours
One of the ways in which parents attempted to cope was through learning to manage their children's challenging behaviours (Duchene, 2015; Berhane, 2016). In studies by both Duchene (2015) and Berhane (2016), parents attempted to manage these behaviours by providing their children with schedules and routines, as they found that these strategies minimised the occurrence of adverse behaviours. Another way of coping was for parents to adjust their expectations of their children and how they behaved (Chao et al., 2017).

A way to prevent difficult behaviours, and thereby enable parents to cope, was to provide children with access to appropriate intervention strategies (Corcoran, Berry & Hill, 2015). However, gaining access to appropriate intervention strategies was found to be somewhat of a challenge for parents (Corcoran, Berry & Hill, 2015). Reasons for this included parents not being aware of all of the resources available to them, treatment options being located too far away from where they live, and long waiting lists to access treatment (Chirwa, 2012; Corcoran, Berry & Hill, 2015; DePape & Lindsay, 2015; Berhane, 2016).

Another way in which parents have been found to cope with their child's challenging behaviours and needs was to remain flexible within their everyday routines (Schaaf, Toth-Cohen, Johnson, Outten & Benevides, 2011), The main areas where parents felt the need for flexibility was with their work schedules and daily routines, whether at home or elsewhere (Schaaf et al., 2011). The need to be able to adjust to the child's needs was critical for these parents (Schaaf et al., 2011). Flexibility was also found to be one of the key aspects of resilient families in a South African study that looked at resilience in families with a child living with ASD (Greeff & Van Der Walt, 2010).

2.2.4.4. Personal growth

One of the ways in which parents were found to cope was through personal growth (Corcoran, Berry & Hill, 2015). One of the most common aspects of growth was that of patience, which has been found in numerous studies (Corcoran, Berry & Hill, 2015; DePape & Lindsay, 2015; Duchene, 2015; Berhane, 2016; Burrell, Ives & Unwin, 2017). Other aspects of growth have included an increase in levels of tolerance and a decrease in judgement towards others (Corcoran, Berry & Hill, 2015; DePape & Lindsay, 2015; Berhane, 2016; Burrell, Ives & Unwin, 2017), an increase in compassion and less of a focus on trivial issues (Marciano, Drasgow & Carlson, 2015), an increase in gratitude, and an increase in the ability to cope with adversity (Corcoran, Berry & Hill, 2015).

Chao et al. (2017) found that one form of coping was for parents to adjust their expectations of their child. Chao et al. (2017) found that adjusting expectations led to a new sense of hope and vision for the future. This included focusing more on the child's capabilities, which was shown to increase parents' abilities to cope with various stressors (Chao et al., 2017). The adjusting of expectations was also found in numerous other studies (Tadesse, 2014; Duchene, 2015; Burrell, Ives & Unwin, 2017).

2.3. Theoretical Framework

The transactional model of stress and coping (Folkman & Lazarus, 1980), as well as resiliency theory (Greene, Galambos & Lee, 2004), were the theoretical frameworks underpinning this study.

2.3.1. Transactional model of stress and coping

Folkman and Lazarus (1980) developed the transactional model of stress and coping in an attempt to explain the dynamics of stress. Through this model, Folkman and Lazarus (1980) explained that when people are faced with a situation, they cognitively appraise and evaluate whether the situation poses a threat to themselves. They purported that there are three possible types of threats that people face, namely: previous harm or loss, potential harm or loss in the future, or having to face a challenge that one needs to master (Folkman & Lazarus, 1980). They called this *primary appraisal* (Folkman & Lazarus, 1980).

Once an individual goes through the process of *primary appraisal*, they cognitively appraise whether they have the resources needed to cope effectively with the threat. This is known as *secondary appraisal* (Folkman & Lazarus, 1980).

The ability to cope consists of the management of an individual's relationship with their environment, which can also be referred to as their resources (Folkman & Lazarus, 1980). This relationship regulates stressful emotions with regard to the situations people face (Folkman & Lazarus, 1980). An individual's coping strategies can also change over time, either increasing or decreasing in effectiveness (Folkman & Lazarus, 1980). As a result of this fluidity, the person's relationship with their environment is seen to be transactional, as they affect one another (Folkman & Lazarus, 1980).

In this study, the transactional model of stress and coping (Folkman & Lazarus, 1980) provided a lens through which the stressors related to caring for a child living with ASD could be viewed and understood, especially as to why they were seen as being stressors in the first place. Furthermore, through this model parents' coping strategies could be understood as it explained how parents appraised whether or not they believed they had the resources needed to cope with these stressors.

2.3.2. Resiliency theory

In their development of resiliency theory, Greene, Galambos and Lee (2004) defined resiliency as peoples' ability to successfully face, and overcome, adversity. According to Greene, Galambos and Lee (2004), resiliency is the result of *internal protective factors*, such as people's attitudes or religion, as well as *external protective factors*, such as family support or a sense of community. These factors would then determine a person's ability to remain resilient in the face of adversity (Greene, Galambos & Lee, 2004). It could therefore be said that a person's ability to be resilient in the face of difficulties is a result of the strengths and protective factors evident in their lives (Greene, Galambos & Lee, 2004). While some people are able to face difficulties with success and others are not, Greene, Galambos and Lee (2004) stated that resiliency can develop over time as people gain access to more resources, meaning that people can increase their ability to succeed when faced with difficulties.

Resiliency theory (Greene, Galambos & Lee, 2004) adds to our understanding of Folkman and Lazarus's (1980) transactional model of stress and coping as it provides in-depth insight into secondary appraisal, as described by Folkman and Lazarus (1980), and utilized by parents with children living with ASD. Resiliency theory allowed for the assessing of respondents' perceived internal and external protective factors, which might have impacted on their perception as to whether or not they had sufficient coping mechanisms available to them.

In discussing the implications of resiliency theory for social work practice, Green, Galambos and Lee (2004) stated that, due to social work's strengths-based approach, social workers need to assess their clients' levels of resilience and include this in intervention planning, as well as promote increased resilience both in terms of the client's internal and external protective factors. Tong (2011) believed that if social workers enabled and empowered their clients to use their strengths and resources to cope, they would lessen the degree of the adversities they faced as a result. This was echoed in South African research conducted by Van Breda (2018), who said that social workers could not merely look at the problems their clients were facing, but needed to consider their clients' strengths as well, especially if their clients were to succeed.

Family resilience has been found to be highly beneficial for parents caring for children living with ASD within a South African context, especially as this population has been found to experience a variety of challenges (Greeff & Van Der Walt, 2010; Simelane, 2015). It has been found that resilient families of this nature are better able to cope with the challenges that they face (Simelane, 2015). In turn, this is beneficial for the well-being of children within South Africa who are living with ASD, as well as the ability for their families to function successfully (Greeff & Van Der Walt, 2010).

2.4. Policy and Legislation

2.4.1. The National Integrated Early Childhood Development Policy

The National Integrated Early Childhood Development (ECD) policy was developed to ensure that children within South Africa are given equal access to developmental services (Department of Social Development [DSD], 2015). One of the gaps in policy and legislation within South Africa is that there has not been specific mention of ASD, and it is therefore assumed that ASD is incorporated within the legislation and policy that applies to those living with a disability within South Africa. According to the ECD policy, children living with a disability in South Africa are seen as being vulnerable, and have therefore been prioritised under ECD as a result (DSD, 2015). The policy states that ECD caters for children from birth to the year in which they attend formal schooling, and that these years are important as this is when developmental milestones are reached (DSD, 2015). The policy reported that no funding had been provided for ECD programmes for vulnerable children before the policy's implementation (DSD, 2015). The policy states that priority should be given to developing, funding and implementing programmes for vulnerable children, and that barriers to accessing these programmes should be addressed (DSD, 2015). This policy is paramount, as its implementation would meet the needs of early care and education for children living with a disability, and, by implication, those living with ASD in South Africa. With this said, it must be stated that there is a lack of resources and infrastructure for these programmes within South Africa, leading to the inequality of treatment for those needing early care and intervention. However, living with ASD in South Africa. As a result of this policy, a few specific programmes have been implemented by DSD as a response to the need for services for children living with ASD, especially as ASD has been recognised as being a disability (DSD, 2013). Although this policy could increase the chances of children being diagnosed earlier with ASD and could ensure they got the care that they needed during these formative years, the policy only caters for ECD and therefore does not cover the needs of children who have started formal schooling.

2.4.2. The Children's Amendment Act

The Children's Act, No. 38 of 2005, as amended (2010) outlines the rights of all children in South Africa, so as to ensure that they are adequately cared for and protected. This act provides a framework within which social services are to be provided for children living within South Africa, and as a result, directly relates to social work practice. This act is inclusive, as, in the interpretation of terms, the care of a child includes the accommodation of their special needs (*Children's Act, No. 38 of 2005, as amended,* 2010). There are numerous sections within the act that speak specifically to children living with a disability (*Children's Act, No. 38 of 2005, as amended,* 2010). Whilst the act does not specifically define what living with a disability encompasses, one might place ASD under this category, as children living with ASD have various special needs over and above children who do not live with ASD. As a result of the inclusivity of the act, ASD is not specifically mentioned.

One of the main objectives of the act is that the special needs of children living with disabilities are recognised (*Children's Act, No. 38 of 2005, as amended,* 2010). With regard to the general principles of the act, section 6(2)(d) states that children need to be protected from unfair discrimination, which includes not being discriminated against due to any disability that they might be living with (*Children's Act, No. 38 of 2005, as amended,* 2010). It goes on further to state that, as part of the general principles of the act, a child's disability needs to be recognised, and their environment needs to cater to their special needs (*Children's Act, No. 38 of 2005, as amended,* 2010). The standard with regard to acting in the best interests of the child states that any disability must be taken into consideration when acting in the child's best interests (*Children's Act, No. 38 of 2005, as amended,* 2010).

The most pertinent section with regard to disability is section 11, which states that consideration must be given for children with disabilities with regard to: their care; their ability to participate in various activities, including education; ensuring their dignity and independence; and providing support services to these children and their caregivers (*Children's Act, No. 38 of 2005, as amended,* 2010). With regard to education, the act recognises that every child, including those living with a disability, have the right to education (*Children's Act, No. 38 of 2005, as amended,* 2010). Additionally, the national norms and standards in S94 (3) with regard to ECD also states that ECD programmes must cater to children living with a disability, as well as any other special needs (*Children's Act, No. 38 of 2005, as amended,* 2010).

Despite the amendments that have been added to *The Children's Act of 2005* (2007), there are still numerous gaps with regard to children living with disabilities. As a result, the *Children's Amendment Bill, No. 244* (2019) is currently being tabled, which, once enacted, will speak to the necessity for, and implementation of, a national strategy with regard to increasing the provision of services to, and meeting the needs of, children with disabilities in South Africa (DSD, 2019). The bill states that this national strategy must include ECD, rehabilitation services and support to children with disabilities (DSD, 2019). It also outlines the need for a wider spread of drop-in centres throughout South Africa, where children with disabilities are catered for (DSD, 2019).

2.5. Conclusion

This chapter presented a review of the literature, key theoretical models, and policy and legislation relevant to the study. By reviewing the literature, it was evident that being a parent of a child living with ASD is complex and includes a variety of experiences, many of which can become stressors. As a result, various coping mechanisms were found to be essential in order to build up resilience and to decrease one's stress levels, as were various forms of formal and informal support. However, for some parents, there seemed to be barriers to being able to utilise all of these coping mechanisms.

Chapter Three - Methodology

3.1. Introduction

This chapter outlines the research methodology used in the study. It begins by looking at the research design, and then moves on to sampling, followed by data collection and analysis.

3.2. Research Design

This study utilised a qualitative research design. A qualitative design is geared towards describing and exploring people's perspectives (Babbie & Mouton, 2001). The main goal of qualitative research is therefore to explore and understand human behaviour (Babbie & Mouton, 2001). This method was ideal for this study, as the study sought to gain an understanding of the parents' world, and their personal and subjective experiences of caring for a child living with ASD.

Furthermore, a qualitative research design is an emergent research process that unfolds with time, meaning that the research process can shift as the study goes on (Creswell, 2014). This process allowed the researcher to remain flexible while data was collected and findings emerged, allowing for the full exploration of the topic.

3.3. Population and Sampling

A study population is a group of people with a specific set of characteristics that encompasses the total group from which respondents are drawn (De Vos et al., 2011). The population of this study was South African parents who were the primary caregivers of children living with ASD. The size of the study population was unknown.

3.3.1. Sampling technique

Non-probability sampling is used when the total study population is unknown (Babbie & Mouton, 2001). In this study, non-probability sampling was used because the borders of the population of parents caring for a child living with ASD within South Africa was difficult to define, and was therefore difficult to access. More specifically, the study used a combination of two types of non-probability sampling, namely: purposive and snowball sampling.

Purposive sampling consists of selecting respondents based on what is known about the population, as well as the purpose of the study (Babbie & Mouton, 2001). The researcher uses their own judgement in selecting respondents based on their knowledge of the population (De Vos et al., 2011). A purposive sampling technique was best suited for this study, as it allowed the researcher to select a sample that had the best knowledge of the subject being researched. This sample consisted of parents of children living with ASD within South Africa. With knowledge on the topic, the researcher decided on inclusion criteria, as outlined below, so that the best respondents were selected for the study.

The researcher only found nine respondents through purposive sampling. As a result, snowball sampling was then utilised to find more respondents. Snowball sampling consists of asking respondents to recommend other people who could be potential respondents (Babbie & Mouton, 2001). Snowball sampling is beneficial as it allows the researcher to find respondents who are otherwise difficult to locate (Babbie & Mouton, 2001). By utilising snowball sampling in this study, the researcher gained an additional 11 respondents.

3.3.2. Sampling characteristics

The 20 respondents interviewed were selected according to specific inclusion criteria. All respondents were the primary care giver of a child living with ASD. The child had received an official diagnosis and the respondent had been the primary caregiver since before the ASD diagnostic process begun. Only the parent who spent the most time with the child was selected. There was initially no sampling criteria with regards to their race, gender or age, but unintentionally all 20 respondents were female, as only mothers volunteered to participate in the study. All respondents were from South Africa and resided in Cape Town, Johannesburg or Durban. Their age, race, income, and marital statuses varied.

3.3.3. Sampling procedure

Various parental support groups, ASD related organisations, and special needs schools that catered for children living with ASD in Cape Town were contacted. Contact was first made telephonically, and was then followed up with an email. These included an explanation of the study and a request to put the researcher in touch with potential respondents that utilised their services. In communicating with these organisations, the researcher specified the sampling criteria for respondents. Once permission was granted for the researcher to be put in touch with possible respondents, the organisations were asked to approach the recipients of their services themselves to offer them the chance to participate in this study. The organisations then made a request to these parents on the researcher's behalf in order to maintain the privacy and anonymity of the recipients of their services. The researcher's contact details were given to potential respondents by the organisation, and those willing to participate contacted the researcher directly.

After contacting numerous organisations, only nine respondents volunteered. It was at this point that the researcher asked those respondents who had already been interviewed if they knew of others who might be interested and willing to participate. Respondents then passed on the researcher's contact details to prospective respondents, and those who were willing to participate contacted the researcher directly.

Once potential respondents contacted the researcher, the researcher explained the study and clarified the sampling criteria with them both telephonically and via email. The researcher also emailed the consent form so that potential respondents could read through it and ask any questions that they might have. Once a potential respondent decided they would like to take part, the respondent and the researcher set up a date, time, and place where the interview would occur.

3.4. Data Collection

3.4.1. Data collection method

Data was collected through the use of semi-structured one-on-one interviews. One-on-one interviews involve asking respondents questions in a verbal manner and recording their answers to these questions (De Vos et al., 2011). Semi-structured interview questions are pre-determined, but open-ended (De Vos et al., 2011). This approach, when used with respondents willing to cooperate and share truthfully, provides the most in-depth data with regard to respondents' perceptions, while remaining flexible and ensuring their privacy (De Vos et al., 2011). This approach was beneficial to the study as the topic was of a sensitive nature. This gave respondents the space to share and the researcher the flexibility to find out more about what respondents had said. This was important as the study was exploratory and little research had been done on the topic before. The ability to be flexible gave the researcher the opportunity to ascertain rich data as it became evident during the interview.

Interviews were conducted either face-to-face or over Skype. Respondents from Cape Town were interviewed face-to-face, while respondents from Johannesburg and Durban were interviewed via Skype. Skype is a Voice over Internet Protocol (VoIP) that gives researchers the ability to interview respondents in a different location from the researcher (Iacono, Symonds & Brown, 2016). This is advantageous, as it increases the possibility of who the researcher can interview (Iacono, Symonds & Brown, 2016). According to Deakin and Wakefield (2013), the use of Skype can increase the willingness of potential respondents to participate in research due to the convenience that Skype affords, both due to time and the flexibility it allows.

Whilst Iacono, Symonds and Brown (2016) found that Skype interviews are a good and viable alternative to face-to-face interviews within the data collection process, they also warned that Skype could affect the ability to establish rapport and read non-verbal communication. However, in a study conducted by Deakin and Wakefield (2013), it was found that in many cases the rapport built over Skype could be just as good as the rapport built when face-to-face.

Within this study, when respondents were interviewed over Skype, the researcher gave them the option to have the video function on or off. According to Sullivan (2012), the video function on Skype can mimic some of the interactions that occur when conducting a face-to-face interview, which could be beneficial for data collection. However, Deakin and Wakefield (2013) found that utilising the video function could also lead to respondents feeling uneasy and anxious, and therefore found that giving respondents the option could be beneficial.

According to Deakin and Wakefield (2013), using Skype without the video function resembles that of a telephonic interview. Like the research on the use of Skype, Farooq and de Villiers (2017) found that telephonic interviews could hinder the establishing of rapport between interviewer and interviewee, however, they also found that there was an increase in the likelihood of participation in a study due to the advantages of saving on both time and money by opting to do telephonic, rather than face-to-face, interviews. Telephonic interviews were also experienced as less intrusive, allowing respondents to feel more comfortable when interviewed (Farooq & de Villiers, 2017). The researcher made it clear to those who did not live in Cape Town that their interview would need to be telephonic before they opted in.

A qualitative research design stipulates that data should be collected in a natural setting to increase comfort (Creswell, 2014). Interviewing respondents within a space that felt natural to them was ideal for this study, as it facilitated a setting in which parents could share their personal experiences and felt comfortable while doing so. Furthermore, interviewing in a private setting ensures confidentiality and privacy (De Vos et al., 2011). With respondents who were interviewed in person, this setting occurred in a private space of respondents' choosing, where they felt most comfortable, such as their home. Respondents who were interviewed telephonically planned the time of the interview in accordance with a time when they could be in a place they felt was both private and comfortable for them. According to Babbie and Mouton (2001), this could be an advantage for respondents who are interviewed telephonically, as they can be interviewed in a more comfortable space they would not usually allow an interviewer into. Most respondents opted to be interviewed in their own homes.

3.4.2. Data collection instrument
In this study, a semi-structured interview schedule (Appendix B) was used when interviewing. An interview schedule is a predetermined set of questions that serves to guide the interview (De Vos et al., 2011). Questions need to be brief, specific and clear, and need to be designed in a way that elicits the information that is sought, while keeping the interview on track (De Vos et al., 2011). In this study, the formulation of questions was led by the research objectives and theoretical framework. It also included demographic questions in the beginning of the interview, and questions were ordered from easy to more emotionally difficult. The schedule ensures that the areas of interest are covered, and allows flexibility to jump back and forth between questions (De Vos et al., 2011).

The interview schedule enables the researcher to take into account respondents' non-verbal cues, and allows the data collection process to be more personal (De Vos et al., 2011). While the researcher noted as many non-verbal cues as possible, it must be noted that for those who were interviewed over Skype without the video function, the entirety of their non-verbal cues were unable to be observed. This potential limitation was construed by Mealer and Jones (2014). Whilst this could have affected the richness of data gathered,

Babbie and Mouton (2001) found that respondents are often more honest telephonically as they do not have eye contact with the interviewer and feelings of judgement are decreased as a result.

The interview schedule was piloted with two respondents. Piloting the interview schedule allows the researcher to refine the questions before interviewing respondents (De Vos et al., 2011). This ensures clarity and that the necessary information is attained (De Vos et al., 2011). This is important, as the way in which each question is worded affects how respondents answer (De Vos et al., 2011). In this study, the data from the pilot interviews was not included in the findings as the researcher refined and adjusted the order of questions thereafter.

3.4.3. Data collection apparatus

A digital recorder was used to record the interviews, with the respondents' informed consent. A recorder provides a full record of each interview and ensures that the researcher can focus on the interview process, instead of trying to remember or write down everything said (De Vos et al., 2011). To ensure appropriate informed consent, information about the recording of the interviews was included in the consent form. Once the interview was complete, the researcher transferred the audio file from the recording device into a password-protected file on a computer, and deleted the original audio file to ensure confidentiality.

During interviews digital recorders need to be placed so that they are not in the eye line of respondents so that respondents are not distracted and do not withdraw from the process as a result (De Vos et al., 2011). In this study, the researcher adhered to this advice when conducting face-to-face interviews, as well as when using the camera function on Skype.

Besides recording, note taking is advised as non-verbal cues and any impressions that are picked up on during interviews should be noted for data collection purposes (De Vos et al., 2011). In this study, notes of various nuances were taken during and immediately after the interview.

3.5. Data Analysis

The data was analysed according to Tesch's eight steps (1990).

- The first step involves gaining a clear, big picture of what the researcher has found (Tesch, 1990). This was done by printing all the transcriptions, reading through them, and then noting any big picture ideas that came to mind.

- Once the researcher has a clear picture of the data as a whole, the next step is to read through each transcription again and note the different topics that emerge (Tesch, 1990). The researcher went through one document at a time in order of when the interviews took place. At this stage, the researcher could begin to see various categories and sub-categories emerging.

- The third step is to cluster the different topics that emerge and then to go through a few transcriptions at a time to compare and connect topics so that they begin to form clusters (Tesch, 1990). The researcher went through four transcriptions at a time to note and cluster topics that related to one another.

- Once topics are clustered, they need to be abbreviated (Tesch, 1990). The first four documents were read through once again and abbreviations were noted in the appropriate margins. According to Tesch (1990), this determines the relevance of each topic that has been noted in the previous step.

- The fifth step of data analysis is to create categories out of the themes that have emerged (Tesch, 1990). Categories that relate to one another are then grouped (Tesch, 1990). The researcher wrote down all of the topics that had emerged into one list, and then grouped them in different ways until she felt that the themes were in the right groupings.

- Once links have been made, the next step is to abbreviate the categories and make final decisions of the abbreviations (Tesch, 1990).

- The seventh step is to conduct an initial analysis on the content of each transcription, and to identify and summarise the findings under each category (Tesch, 1990). Similarities, differences, confusions, and potential missing information are then identified (Tesch, 1990). At this point, the researcher switched from using paper and pen, and began to work electronically. For this study, the content was analysed with the help of Nvivo, a computer-based programme. Nvivo is said to allow for more time efficiency, and to make sorting and reorganising data easier (Leech & Onwuegbuzie, 2011). The researcher went through each transcription and highlighted and categorised each idea that was shared into electronic categories and sub-categories.

- The final step of data analysis is to repeat the process for the remaining data (Tesch, 1990). At times this led to the need to recode existing data, as some of the coding became redundant. This was made easier through the use of Nvivo, as it was easy to recode data within the programme. Once the researcher had completed this process with all 20 transcriptions, the researcher used the programme to create individual documents that grouped all of the data for each category and subcategory together. This made it easier to write up the findings of the study as data from each category and subcategory was in one document. This final step ensures that the findings are in line with the purpose of the research (Tesch, 1990).

3.6. Data Verification

Data verification addresses the validity and reliability of a study, so that it can be ensured that the study's findings are trustworthy (Lincoln & Guba, 1985). Data verification was considered with regard to credibility, transferability, dependability, and confirmability.

3.6.1. Credibility

Credibility refers to ensuring that the findings reflect what respondents have shared (Lincoln & Guba, 1985). One way of ensuring that findings are credible is to ensure that data saturation has occurred before the data collection process comes to an end (Lincoln & Guba, 1985). This was adhered to in this study, as the researcher interviewed enough respondents that no new information was being provided that had not been provided before. Credibility can be further ensured by having the resources needed to document what is shared during interviews (Lincoln & Guba, 1985). In this study, interviews were recorded with the respondents' consent and were thereafter transcribed, so as to have a true and accurate account of what the respondents shared without the risk of relying on the researcher's memory. One of the resources that Lincoln and Guba (1985) referred to was having a method in which to note important non-verbal communication while interviewing respondents. The researcher noted important non-verbal communication straight after each interview, so as to have an accurate record of this that could be used once data analysis occurred.

3.6.2. Transferability

Transferability is the ability to transfer the study's findings on to other members of the study population, and is therefore the extent to which these findings can be generalised to others (Lincoln & Guba, 1985). One strategy that can be used to ensure transferability is to provide rich descriptions of the study sample (Lincoln & Guba, 1985). This study provided rich descriptions within the sampling characteristics above and in the demographics, as presented in Chapter Four. Another strategy is to ensure that findings are presented in the context in which they are given (Lincoln & Guba, 1985). This study ensured that the context in which information was given was conveyed within the presentation of findings and conclusions of this paper. Transferability can also be ensured through the use of purposive sampling whereby the researcher ensures that a range of respondents are chosen so as to include differing aspects of the study population (Lincoln & Guba, 1985). In this study, purposive sampling was only used for the first nine respondents, and was then replaced with snowball sampling in an effort to increase the size of the research sample. Due to this, the transferability of the study might have been affected, due to respondents referring others who are similar to them. The similarities of respondents with regard to gender and socioeconomic status is an example of this, and is referred to in the limitations below.

3.6.3. Dependability

The dependability of a study is the ability for the study to be repeated with similar subjects within similar contexts and to conclude with similar findings (Lincoln & Guba, 1985). According to Lincoln and Giba (1985) a study is found to be dependable through the same techniques as those employed in ensuring credibility. Examples of these techniques include ensuring data saturation has taken place and and that the researcher has the resources needed to adequately document the interviews, both of which were done in this study, as presented above. A further way of ensuring dependability is to attain an auditor who can check the documents that were used to analyse the data and conclude findings (Lincoln & Guba, 1985). While this study did not make use of an auditor, the researcher was held accountable to the researcher's supervisor, which may have assisted in ensuring the dependability of this study.

3.6.4. Confirmability

Confirmability refers to the objectivity of the study's findings, and the absence of bias in this regard (Lincoln & Guba, 1985). This can be achieved through a *confirmability audit trail*, which Lincoln and Guba (1985) suggested should involve reviewing the data to ensure that it is objectively sound. This includes: reviewing the study's raw data; documents pertaining to the reduction and analysis of data; documents pertaining to the synthesis of the data analysis, and therefore the reconstruction of data; all notes, including those used for process and analysis; and the information used to develop the instrument that collected data (Lincoln & Guba, 1985). In this study, the researcher and the researcher's supervisor reviewed the data multiple times to ensure that it was objective and that there was an absence of bias. The researcher also ensured reflexivity, as referred to below, so as to ensure that the researcher's own perceptions did not taint the objetivity of the data.

3.7. Reflexivity

Reflexivity refers to the researcher reflecting on and understanding their own perceptions (De Vos et al., 2011). This is important as the researcher needs to be aware of the ways in which their perceptions might have an impact on the findings of the research (Creswell, 2014). The researcher needs to guard against this by remaining objective when collecting and interpreting data (Creswell, 2014).

In this study, the researcher was a friend of a couple whose son had been diagnosed with ASD. This friendship led to the researcher having witnessed some of the difficulties that parents might face as a result of an ASD diagnosis. Hence, there is a strong emotional connection to this area of study. These emotions included sadness towards the difficulties that parents in the study had faced as a result of their child's ASD, and anger towards those who had stigmatised them and misunderstood their difficulties. Due to being aware of this emotional connection to the topic of the study, the researcher ensured she remained neutral and unbiased during the data collection and interpretation process, so as not to filter the findings through her own judgement and bias.

Furthermore, the researcher is a registered Social Worker, and due to her empathy for parents who have children living with ASD, she needed to ensure not to fall into a therapeutic role during the data collection process. This was avoided by using an interview schedule so as not to divert to asking questions that might be unnecessary for the purposes of this study. The researcher ensured that she remained within the role of researcher and did not default to a therapeutic role. The researcher also referred respondents for additional support, if deemed necessary, to ensure that she remained in the role of researcher.

3.8. Limitations

It is important to acknowledge any limitations that the study might have, as well as any that might occur during the research process (De Vos et al., 2011).

It was difficult to find respondents for this study, especially when using purposive sampling. This could have been due to a myriad of reasons, including respondents not having the time to be interviewed, especially considering the stressors faced by these parents, or not wanting to share their struggles with someone they did not know. The exact reasons why potential respondents did not volunteer to participate in this study were not explored. To overcome the limitation of not having enough respondents, the sampling method was shifted to snowball sampling, which allowed for the number of respondents needed in this study so that data saturation could occur.

In this study, the topic could have been emotive for respondents, which might have led to respondents not being open and honest. Respondents might have also feared judgement or felt anxious due to needing to be vulnerable, and not wanted to share certain aspects of their experiences. The researcher attempted to make the interview feel emotionally safe for respondents by ensuring their privacy and comfort, and by explaining the confidentiality agreement with them to mitigate this limitation as much as possible. Rapport was also built during the interviews so that respondents felt more comfortable and less judged. Respondents gave the impression that they felt comfortable while being interviewed, and shared a lot of their experiences, however, the researcher could not be sure that respondents were fully open and honest.

Another possible limitation was the lack of diversity with regard to the population sample that the findings represented. Firstly, mothers were the only parents who were interviewed and therefore the perceptions of fathers were not captured. Secondly, most respondents seemed to come from more affluent circumstances. Resultantly, the results of this study could be skewed towards more affluent South African mothers within the total study population. One of the recommendations of this study is that further research is conducted on this study population, especially regarding the experiences of fathers and parents of varying socioeconomic standings.

3.9. Conclusion

In conclusion, this study consisted of a qualitative research design. Non-probability sampling was used and consisted of both purposive and snowball sampling. Data was collected via semi-structured one-on-one interviews and was analysed in line with Tesch's (1990) eight steps. The researcher verified the data, remained reflexive, and aimed to mitigate potential limitations during the research process where possible.

Chapter Four – Findings

4.1. Introduction

This chapter begins by providing a demographic profile of the respondents, followed by the framework of analysis, and finally a presentation of the findings. Findings emerged in relation to the three objectives that guided the study.

4.2. Demographic Profile of Respondents

Table 1: Demographic Profile of Respondents

Res-pond-ent	Gender	Age	Race	City of residence	Employ-ment status	Child depen-dents	Age of child at time of diagnosis	Years since diagnosis
1	Female	39	White	Cape Town	Full-time	2	2	1
2	Female	50	White	Cape Town	Part-time	2	4	11
3	Female	31	Indian	Cape Town	Not seeking	2	1	7
4	Female	37	Black	Cape Town	Full-time	2	2	4
5	Female	40	Coloured	Cape Town	Full-time	2	2; 10*	12; 2
6	Female	46	White	Cape Town	Not seeking	2	4	6
7	Female	37	Indian	Cape Town	Not seeking	3	5	1
8	Female	44	White	Johannesburg	Full-time	2	5	2
9	Female	46	White	Durban	Part-time	2	2	7
10	Female	48	White	Johannesburg	Full-time	1	3	4
11	Female	31	White	Johannesburg	Full-time	1	2	3
12	Female	41	White	Cape Town	Not seeking	5	8	2
13	Female	39	White	Johannesburg	Full-time	1	3	2
14	Female	43	White	Johannesburg	Full-time	1	5	3
15	Female	34	White	Johannesburg	Job seeking	2	2	2
16	Female	46	Black	Johannesburg	Full-time	1	2	1
17	Female	51	White	Cape Town	Full-time	2	3	8
18	Female	52	White	Johannesburg	Full-time	2	10	2
19	Female	48	White	Cape Town	Full-time	3	2	6
20	Female	46	Coloured	Cape Town	Not seeking	2	3	7

---

* This reflects the respective ages of Respondent 5's two children diagnosed with ASD

Table 1 shows the demographic profile of the 20 respondents. All respondents were female and ranged from 31 to 51 years of age. Two respondents identified their race as Black, two as Indian, two as Coloured, and 14 as White.

At the time of the study, 11 respondents lived in Cape Town, eight lived in Johannesburg, and one lived in Durban. When asked about their employment status, 12 respondents reported being employed full-time, while two were employed part-time, five were not currently looking for employment, and one was job-seeking.

When it came to the number of child dependents each respondent cared for, five respondents had one dependent, while 12 respondents had two, two respondents had three, and one respondent had five. Only one respondent had two children diagnosed with ASD, and they were diagnosed at ages 2 and 10 respectively. The rest of the respondents had only one child diagnosed with ASD.

Respondents were asked at what age their children were diagnosed. One child was diagnosed at 1 years old, while eight were at the age of 2, four at the age of 3, two at the age of 4, three at the age of 5, one at the age of 8, and two at the age of 10. The most prevalent age for diagnosis for respondents' children was 2 years old. Amongst the respondents' children, all except three were diagnosed before they turned 6 years old. With regard to the number of years since the children of the respondents were diagnosed, three children had received a diagnosis one year prior to the time of the interview, while six were two years prior, two were three years prior, two were four years prior, two were six years prior, three were seven years prior, one was eight years prior, one was 11 years prior, and one was 12 years prior.

The findings of the study will now be presented in the form of a framework of analysis, followed by a presentation of the findings.

4.3. Framework of Analysis

Table 2: Framework of Analysis

Themes	Categories	Subcategories
Stressors faced by parents	Stressors related to the child's ASD symptoms	The child's difficult behaviours
		The struggle to communicate with their child
		Anxiety experienced by parents as a result of caring for a child living with ASD
	Practicalities of caring for a child living with ASD	Multiple HCPs in diagnosis journey
		The cost of care and interventions
		Finding an appropriate school
	Stressors related to parents' own emotions	Emotional responses when child was diagnosed
		Hurt and difficulties from others' lack of understanding of ASD
		Concerns about their child's future
Coping mechanisms	Psychological forms of coping	Adjusting expectations and hopes for their child's future
		Acceptance of the child with the diagnosis
		Personal growth of the parent
	Practical ways of coping	Management of their child's difficult behaviours
		Utilisation of a blend of interventions from HCPS and other professionals
		Educating themselves on ASD
		Educating others on ASD
Support mechanisms	Support from family	
	Informal support from other parents	

4.4. Presentation of Findings

The findings of the study will be discussed under the headings of the above framework.

4.4.1. Stressors faced by parents

Three categories emerged in relation to the first objective of the study, which was to explore the stressors faced by parents of children living with ASD. As defined by Folkman and Lazarus (1980) in their transactional model of stress and coping, stressors are events that could lead, or have led, to harm or loss, or that have presented a challenge. In this study, the stressors reported to have been experienced by respondents are presented under three main categories, namely: stressors related to the child's ASD symptoms, the practicalities of parenting a child living with ASD, and the parents' own emotions. These categories, as well as their subcategories, will be presented below.

4.4.1.1. Stressors related to the child's ASD symptoms

Three subcategories were found to pertain to the stressors specifically related to respondents' interactions with their child's ASD symptoms. These subcategories were: dealing with the child's difficult behaviours, the struggle to communicate with their child, and the parent's anxiety due to caring for a child living with ASD. These stressors were both related to what Folkman and Lazarus (1980) saw as events that presented a challenge.

4.4.1.1.1. The child's difficult behaviours

All respondents spoke about the challenges they face in dealing with the difficult behaviours that their children display. These included challenges such as inappropriate social behaviours, unpredictability, and rigidity.

She was incredibly demanding and incredibly difficult... She has a communication delay, sensory issues, [and] rigid behaviour... [As a] baby, she literally never slept. That was a huge problem... when you've got a small child running around for 18 hours without ever sleeping, that's incredibly challenging... [It was] difficult because she was literally always wanting to move, always wanting this deep pressure... The other thing is she's got a lot of anxiety about going out... She doesn't like going to different places that she doesn't know... she's always on the move and obviously the safety considerations around autistic children... No sense of fear... And then very rigid ways of being... you must always drive the same route to a certain place. If you deviate from that route, then she'll have a meltdown. We must all sit in the same place in the house every day... it's very challenging and I think the hardest thing about it is that it's very relentless... I found the unpredictability very unsettling because you just never know what's going to happen... The difficulty with autism is the behavioural issues. (Respondent 10, Female, 48)

He will make noises and he'll start screaming or he'll have fits of laughter... when we're all together and we're talking, he runs off. And he has this habit of taking people's hands or going to give them a hug... when we go to a restaurant, you have to hold both his hands because he'll walk past somebody and grab their drink or eat their chips... He used to touch his private parts in the shop and put his hands in his pants, so you'd have to have control of both hands... But it's a lot harder taking him out in public because of the noises. He draws attention... you avoid social gatherings quite a lot because his behaviour is not acceptable and not everyone understands. (Respondent 20, Female, 46)

Managing their child's difficult behaviours was found to be a challenge for all respondents, and through the examples above one can sense the exasperation that many respondents expressed. The challenges faced can therefore be seen as stressors as found in the studies of Valicenti-McDermott et al. (2015) and Berhane (2016), which found that difficult ASD-related behaviours increased stress levels in parents. These challenges also confirm Shawler and Sullivan's (2015) assertion that the managing of these difficult behaviours is a stressor for parents. Respondents in this study shared some of the strategies they used to manage their child's difficult behaviours. An example of this is trying to control their child's hands while in public, as shared by respondent 20.

Embarrassment was found to be a further stressor, as difficult behaviours were often found to occur in public for the respondents, which Burrell, Ives and Unwin (2017) suggested could compound feelings of frustration, anger, and guilt in parents. Due to the embarrassment experienced, most respondents also spoke about how they avoided being in public as a result of these difficult behaviours, and displayed their frustration when talking about this.

4.4.1.1.2. The struggle to communicate with their child
Most respondents said that one of the difficulties in caring for their children is their struggle to communicate with each other. These respondents further explained that, at times, this struggle to communicate would result in frustration and meltdowns for the child, which further led to this being a stressor for them as parents.

My son struggles to communicate verbally... he isn't able to say in so many words, "Mommy, I am upset because of this..." So he will have more tantrums because he is unable to verbalise that frustration... He is unable to communicate his needs accurately, so when he wants something and he doesn't know the words for that thing, he will shout. He will pick something up and he will throw it on the floor. (Respondent 11, Female, 31)

He can't tell us if he's in pain. It's the communication [that is a challenge at home]. And now he's got ways to try, but it's difficult... He won't tell us when he needs to go [to the toilet], so we have to take him every single hour. (Respondent 15, Female, 34)

She had completely stopped talking... I started to get very worried... The biggest challenge for me is the understanding... at this stage a typical child should be able to have conversations. So for me right now, the challenge is not being able to communicate with her. She doesn't understanding, "stop it," or, "don't do that and don't go there."... Not knowing if she's okay and sometimes when I see her crying she can't tell me what happened. (Respondent 16, Female, 46)

From the above examples, as was the case for the majority of respondents in this study, it can be seen that the realities regarding the struggle to communicate with their children has been experienced as a stressor. This finding further confirms the conclusions of Marciano, Drasgow and Carlson (2015), who found that high levels of stress were found in parents when their children were unable to communicate verbally. Tadesse (2014) found that one possible reason that the struggle to communicate is a stressor for parents is that many children living with ASD are unable to express their needs, leading to frustration. In this study, respondents spoke about the increase in their child's levels of frustration due to this inability to communicate their needs. Furthermore, Valicenti-McDermott et al (2015) also found that children experienced irritability as a result of their struggle to communicate, which could be a challenge for parents. These findings are important, as Kavaliotis (2017) found that high levels of stress could lead to a decrease in resilience and in the ability to cope. This could mean that stressors linked to the struggle to communicate may decrease respondents' ability to cope with adversity.

4.4.1.1.3. Anxiety experienced by parents as a result of caring for a child living with ASD
Most respondents mentioned experiencing anxiety due to caring for a child living with ASD. A common reason for anxiety was due to the need to remain vigilant due to the child's unpredictability and impulsivity.

I now have quite a high level of anxiety, which is something I've never had before... you live in [a state] of always being watchful, always being concerned, always having to make sure that the child hasn't run out in the traffic... You are constantly overwhelmed... I've read studies that say that parenting an autistic child is the equivalent stress of being a combat soldier... I can believe that... it is an unnaturally difficult situation to be in. (Respondent 10, Female, 48)

Sometimes you just feel so drained because you're always constantly busy with him. And I feel like I don't always get to be there as much for my other children as much as I would like to. So it's quite tiring sometimes... And sometimes I am very stressed because he's being difficult. (Respondent 19, Female, 48)

Various studies (Smith et al., 2010; Corcoran, Berry & Hill, 2015; Marciano, Drasgow & Carlson, 2015) have found that caring for a child living with ASD can lead to high levels of anxiety. This concurred with the findings of this study, as most respondents spoke about their anxiety as a result of caring for their children. Tadesse (2014) also found this to be the case, as they found that parents who cared for a child living with ASD were more susceptible to the emotion of anxiety. Seltzer et al. (2010) conducted a study whereby they measured the cortisol levels of mothers who cared for a child living with ASD. They found that the cortisol levels in these mothers was comparable to combat soldiers, people who survived the Holocaust, and those who suffered from post-traumatic stress disorder (Seltzer et al., 2010). This finding is an important one, as it highlights how high the anxiety levels in parents caring for a child living with ASD could be. However, as Whitmore (2016) stated, it is impossible to separate the percentage of a parent's level of stress due to caring for their child's ASD, from their overall level of stress. Therefore, one must not attribute all of the respondents' negative emotions and high levels of stress on caring for their children living with ASD.

4.4.1.2. Practicalities of caring for a child living with ASD

The second set of stressors that was revealed was some of the practicalities for parents of caring for a child living with ASD. These stressors related to what Folkman and Lazarus (1980) referred to as events that present a challenge, as parents found that managing these practicalities challenged them on various levels. The practicalities that respondents shared as being stressful included the need to consult multiple HCPs in the diagnosis journey, the high cost of care and interventions for their child, and finding an appropriate school for their child, among others.

4.4.1.2.1. Multiple HCPs in diagnosis journey

Most respondents had to see multiple HCPs in their journey towards receiving a diagnosis of ASD for their children. Respondents reported that the diagnosis therefore took a considerable amount of time.

And then we started going to the doctors and then from one doctor to another... everyone kept on telling us, "It's not autism, you're crazy!"... "Boys develop late."... The more we said autism, the more they said, "No." And eventually we ended up at an ENT [Ear, Nose and Throat Specialist], who said that he couldn't hear; he probably lost his hearing and needs to go for grommets. [He] went in for the operation, came out 5 minutes later and [the ENT] said, "Sorry, he doesn't need it."... Eventually, in November, he went to the neurologist and he was diagnosed. (Respondent 3, Female, 31)

At 24 months, when she turned 2, I took her to the 'paed' [paediatrician]... then he said... we should first take her for hearing... So I took her to the audiologist and they did all the tests and said her problem was not hearing... maybe she's just delayed in speech so take her for speech therapy... So I went back to her paed and told him I think she's autistic... [He referred] me to a developmental paed... so I called and her appointments were full for so long... She could only see me three months later. I Googled other developmental paeds in JHB and I found one... she was quicker so I went to her and she told me that she would refer me to [another HCP]... She could see that I was a

desperate mother just looking for answers... It took a long time [to get a diagnosis].
(Respondent 16, Female, 46)

Most respondents expressed irritation when they spoke about the need to have appointments with multiple HCPs before their child could receive an official ASD diagnosis. Over and above the frustration that was communicated verbally, respondents who were interviewed in person and over Skype with the use of the video function demonstrated nonverbal cues, for example eye rolls and deep sighs, when speaking on this subject. The need to consult multiple HCPs could therefore be seen as a stressor for respondents. While Crane et al. (2015) found that merely going through the diagnostic process was found to be a challenge for parents, this study found that it was not just going through the diagnostic process that was a challenge, but having to go through multiple HCPs and therefore having a delay in receiving this diagnosis was seen as a stressor. This is similar to DePape and Lindsay's (2015) research, where the delay in receiving a diagnosis was found to be a stressor for parents.

One of the reasons for needing to see multiple HCPs in the diagnosis journey could be due to DePape and Lindsay's (2015) finding that HCPs often have to rule out other possible diagnoses before making a diagnosis of ASD. Respondents reported needing to see multiple HCPs, each with a different specialisation, as a result of needing to rule out other possible diagnoses first, such as hearing loss. It appears, therefore, that ASD's diagnostic process is complex and that this complexity is a stressor for parents.

4.4.1.2.2. The cost of care and interventions
All respondents spoke about the fact that providing the right care and interventions for their children is very expensive. The most common expenses mentioned by respondents included appropriate schooling and interventions needed, as well as the high cost of medication.

So the problem we've found is between the ages of 3 and 6 you don't often find
affordable places that are prepared to look after them... the speech therapist is
expensive, and with him going to [school] we're going to have to cut the speech
therapy... So finances are another stressor for us. (Respondent 1, Female, 39)

It's really expensive. I mean we [spend] almost R10 000 a month [for] medical aid just for the kids and me. It's a lot... The cognitive behavioural therapist is R1 300 an hour, so I'm glad we're only seeing him once a month... [Occupational Therapy] is about R2 000 a month... [Medication] is R500 a month. The psychiatrist is R700 a visit. So it adds up. (Respondent 12, Female, 41)

My research took me to [school's name]... unfortunately I couldn't go there because it was too expensive and I couldn't afford it... so I ended up finding another school for her... but it was also a private school and it was killing me financially. I used all my life's savings... I knew I could only do it for a year... and that is not even talking about the therapies yet, because those are separate. (Respondent 16, Female, 46)

Every respondent spoke about how expensive care and interventions were for their children. Respondents shared how this expense was a challenge for them, which could therefore be seen as being a stressor. This was in accordance with studies that found that parents experienced financial strain due to their child's diagnosis (Centers for Disease Control and Prevention, 2014a; Tadesse, 2014; Kavaliotis, 2017). Moreover, some studies found that reasons for financial strain included high treatment costs and the expense of appropriate schooling (Tadesse, 2014; Berhane, 2016; Hartley et al., 2016; Kavaliotis, 2017).

South African literature emphasised the availability of government grants that parents could access in order to gain financial support (Burrell, Ives & Unwin, 2017). However, these grants were not available to respondents in this study as their household income was too high to qualify. Despite falling outside of the criteria to access these grants, respondents still experienced the cost of care and interventions as being a stressor. This could mean that irrespective of the socioeconomic status of parents caring for a child living with ASD in South Africa, there is a significant financial burden placed on parents due to the high costs associated with providing care for a child living with ASD.

4.4.1.2.3. Finding an appropriate school

Most respondents described the difficulties they had to go through to find an appropriate school for their children, often trying multiple schools before finding the right one. The difficulties that parents went through included moving their children from mainstream schooling to an ASD-focused school, long waiting lists at preferred schools, not agreeing with a school's philosophy on how to educate children living with ASD, a shortage of the kind of schooling that they desired for their children, and not living within a preferred school's catchment area.

There are very few schools who are actually equipped to deal with autistic children, so then you have to start looking for schools and people to help you... A lot of people that I meet report horrendously having to change schools all the time for various reasons. So I think that's very stressful because I think just the change itself is stressful for the child, and then very stressful for the parents because you always have to find a new school, which is more expensive or further away. (Respondent 10, Female, 48)

The first thing that we did [post-diagnosis] was tried to find a specialised school that knew more about autism, had dealt with kids who are autistic, and understood what they needed and how to teach them... So [my child] is now 5 years old. He's been in 5 different schools... [One of the schools was] very clinical. They were all wearing nurses outfits. They were treating the kids as patients instead of kids... [He] was only there for 3 months... Then we found a wonderful little school... but they catered for mental disabilities... Last year we decided to take him out because his peers were starting to tease him because he wasn't communicating... and now we have moved [him]... to another school. (Respondent 11, Female, 31)

I know what kind of school he needs to be at; the fact is that it doesn't exist. And the schools that are available, whether they are mainstream or otherwise, don't actually create an environment in which he can thrive. (Respondent 17, Female, 51)

Finding the right school for their child was found to be a challenge for most respondents. While most respondents found finding the right school to be a challenge, some of these respondents had eventually found an appropriate school for their child, while others had not yet reached that point. The respondents' struggle to find appropriate schooling was not unique, as this was found in various studies (e.g. Rubenstein et al., 2015; Johansson, 2016; Burrell, Ives & Unwin, 2017). These studies found that the main reason for these struggles was that the majority of cost-effective schooling did not cater for children living with ASD-related needs (Rubenstein et al., 2015; Johansson, 2016; Burrell, Ives & Unwin, 2017).

Respondents in this study alluded to the need for parents to advocate for their children to be accepted into their schools of choice, which concurred with the findings of various other studies (Rubenstein et al., 2015; Johansson, 2016; Burrell, Ives & Unwin, 2017). Whilst this was not a trend in this particular study, previous research found that some parents resorted to homeschooling their children to deal with the challenge of finding appropriate schooling (Hurlbutt, 2011; Olatunji, 2014). This might not have been a trend in this study due to the majority of respondents working either full- or part-time, as can be seen in the Demographic Profile of Respondents (Table 1), and therefore not having the time to home-school their children.

4.4.1.3. Stressors related to parents' own emotions

One of the categories that was found under the theme of stressors that were faced by parents was that of stressors related to parents' own emotions. Respondents experienced various emotions as a result of the stressors that they faced. These included: their emotional response when their child was diagnosed, hurt and difficulties due to others' lack of understanding of ASD, and concerns about their child's future.

4.4.1.3.1. Emotional responses when child was diagnosed

Most respondents mentioned that they had experienced negative emotions as a reaction to receiving an official diagnosis of ASD for their child. Negative emotions on receiving the official diagnosis included grief, feelings of loss, sadness, fear, and self-blame.

You are absolutely devastated as a parent... [We were] very sad. I think a lot of grief. Just realising that your child is very different and that their life is not going to be easy... And the loss of this child, who up until this point you think is absolutely 100% healthy and perfect... You suddenly realise... the reality is very different. (Respondent 10, Female, 48)

It was horrible! The first thing that went through my mind was what did I do wrong? Was I the person that gave this to him? It's this fear and threat that there is something that your child has that is going to destroy his life... So I was distraught and depressed because I thought this was something that I gave him. (Respondent 11, Female, 31)

I had immense fear... And that initial diagnosis was hectic. It was kind of earth shattering... And we went through a process of grieving, because we had to grieve the loss of the son we thought we were going to have. (Respondent 15, Female, 34)

The examples above exhibit the negative emotions that most respondents in this study experienced as a result of receiving an ASD diagnosis for their children. Previous studies that were reviewed showed contradictory findings, with some saying parents experienced negative emotion due to getting a diagnosis (Crane et al., 2015; Berhane, 2016; Burrell, Ives & Unwin, 2017; Chao et al., 2017), and others reporting positive emotion (Tadesse, 2014; Corcoran, Berry & Hill, 2015). The findings within this study are in agreement with previous research, by Crane et al. (2015), Berhane (2016), Burrell et al (2017), and Chao et al. (2017), who found that primarily negative emotion was experienced when receiving a diagnosis for one's child. No positive emotions were expressly reported by the respondents, but this might have been due to the fact that prior to asking respondents about their emotional response to their child's diagnosis, respondents had shared their emotions about the process that they went through in obtaining this diagnosis. This process, as reported above, was quite a stressful experience and so asking these questions in this order might have left the respondents focusing and therefore sharing more about their negative rather than positive emotions regarding the diagnosis itself.

Within this study, negative emotions such as grief, loss and sadness were primarily caused by the incongruence between the preconceived ideas that respondents had regarding what it would mean to rear a child, and the lived reality of caring for a child living with ASD. This was found to lead to a period of mourning, whereby they mourned the hopes, dreams and expectations that they had for their child prior to the diagnosis. Previous research has highlighted the loss that many parents experience post-diagnosis, especially due to their change in perception of their child's reality and future (Corcoran, Berry & Hill, 2015; Crane et al., 2015; DePape & Lindsay, 2015; Chao et al., 2017). Seeing the period of mourning as being a stressor is linked to Folkman and Lazarus's (1980) definition of a stressor as being an event that leads to loss.

4.4.1.3.2. Hurt and difficulties from others' lack of understanding of ASD

All respondents spoke about the difficulty of other people not understanding ASD. For respondents, this lack of understanding was apparent with friends and family members, at schools, with HCPs, during interventions, and in public places.

I don't think that there's enough understanding of what autism is... Like people look at you... sometimes you think it would be better if he looked like there was something wrong with him because people would be more accepting... Our friends that do have kids don't understand what's difficult... So I don't think our friends have been as supportive as we were hoping them to be... Maybe the first original reason why I wrote [about ASD] was because I felt like our friends didn't get it and so maybe it was a passive-aggressive way of telling my friends that this is how hard it is. (Respondent 13, Female, 39)

People still hurt us... The hardest part of autism is other people... You do get stared at. You get dirty looks like you're a bad parent. People have said harsh things on an aeroplane when [my child] wouldn't sit down... And I explained [to this woman] that he's got autism and she didn't care. She said, "well, he shouldn't be here then."... Those are the most hurtful [comments], where it's like, "then he doesn't belong here..." That kind of rejection. And it's even more hurtful when it's your child... But it's also close friends and family; the ones who don't say anything to your face but you can feel when they are discussing it... We probably get worse looks because he just looks so normal. (Respondent 14, Female, 43)

This study found that one of the stressors for respondents was other people's lack of understanding of ASD. This finding relates to previous studies that found that there was a lack of understanding of ASD, and that parents faced stigmatisation as a result (Tadesse, 2014; Corcoran, Berry & Hill, 2015; DePape & Lindsay, 2015; Selman et al., 2017). It is interesting to note that some communities had never heard of ASD (Tadesse, 2014), and some languages did not have a word to refer to ASD (Selman et al., 2017). This highlights the lack of knowledge of ASD in many communities, which seemed to be evident in the communities surrounding respondents, and which, therefore, added to the stressors that respondents faced. This might indicate why respondents felt the need to educate others on ASD, however, this will be discussed below regarding the practical ways of coping.

4.4.1.3.3. Concerns about their child's future

Most respondents experienced anxiety or uncertainty with regard to their children's future. The respondents' concerns about their children's future pertained to the parents' mortality, the child's social connectedness, and the child's financial independence.

In terms of emotion, my sadness is: what will his social isolation be like when he's older? And a concern about his lack of financial independence... So my sadness is more for the manner in which he will struggle, possibly in later years... Is he going to grow up and get married? Is he going to work? Is he going to be financially independent? (Respondent 8, Female, 44)

I think the most daunting thing about having a child on the spectrum is you think: what's the future? And I also say to my husband we should be saving money. But we're not. We're just treading water... What happens if [my child] can't look after herself in the future? And what happens when we die? Who's going to look after this child? So I think that's one of the biggest stressors of being the parent of an autistic child... You are constantly worrying about what's going to happen in 20 years time when you're maybe dead... So you think: how is my child going to make it? ... [My child is] always going to be challenged from a social and communication point of view... [As a parent] you are in a constant state of feeling overwhelmed... by all of these issues: by money, the future, and your child... The constant feeling of being out of control and overwhelmed and anxious... I'm even scared to fly now because I'm scared of what's going to happen if the plane crashes. (Respondent 10, Female, 48)

As in the examples above, most respondents verbalised multiple anxieties about their children's futures. This was in line with studies that found that parents experienced a multitude of anxieties in this regard (Tadesse, 2014; DePape & Lindsay, 2015; Berhane, 2016; Burrell, Ives & Unwin, 2017). One of the greatest anxieties for respondents was who would look after their children if something were to happen to them in the future. This echoed existing literature that found that parents were anxious about what would happen to their children if they, as parents, were no longer able to care for their children (Tadesse, 2014; Berhane, 2016). Respondents had concerns about their child's social connectedness, which included their child's ability to form relationships, gain support, and effectively communicate with others in the future. This concern might have also been linked to who would be there for the child if something were to happen to them as parents.

Respondents also experienced anxiety regarding their children's access to finances in the future, which aligned with other studies that found that parents were concerned their children would experience difficulties finding employment and being financially independent (DePape & Lindsay, 2015; Burrell, Ives & Unwin, 2017). In this study, parents had to readjust their future expectations for their children due to ASD. This was similar to literature where, once children were diagnosed with ASD, their parents had to deal with the loss of the dreams that they once had for their children, as they realised that they were most probably no longer realistic (Corcoran, Berry & Hill, 2015; Crane et al., 2015; DePape & Lindsay, 2015).

4.4.2. Coping mechanisms

Two categories emerged in relation to the second objective of the study, which was to explore the coping strategies that parents use in caring for children living with ASD. The development of coping mechanisms seems understandable when taking into account the number of stressors that were exhibited by respondents in the findings above. Two main categories arose from the findings, namely coping mechanisms that were of a psychological nature, and coping mechanisms that were practical. The different coping mechanisms discussed by respondents will be presented under these two categories.

4.4.2.1 Psychological forms of coping

The psychological coping mechanisms that were found in this study included adjusting expectations and hopes for their child's future, accepting the child with their diagnosis, and the personal growth of the parent.

4.4.2.1.1. Adjusting expectations and hopes for their child's future

Most respondents mentioned that, in order to cope, they adjusted their expectations and hopes for their child's future.

I mustn't be too negative because there can be a lot of change and progress... You can't put out there that he'll never go to high school or university because it might change.... My nephew graduated last week and I said to my sister, "I don't know if we're ever going to see that." At this point I'd just be happy if he could communicate with us. My great expectation for now would be just to get him toilet trained. It would be huge in our lives if he could tell us or go by himself to the toilet. (Respondent 1, Female, 39)

I think I just want him to be able to cope on his own; that's the only thing. I don't want him to 'be this' and 'do that' and earn a lot of money, I just want him to be able to function in society. (Respondent 2, Female, 50)

Your parenting skills, the way that you raise your child and the expectations you have for your child. Simple things. Whether it's a sleepover or whether it's more dramatic, like a boyfriend-girlfriend situation, getting married, becoming independent, or having their own job. All of that has to change. (Respondent 17, Female, 51)

Respondents reported needing to adjust the future expectations they had for their children, which was in accordance with previous studies (Tadesse, 2014; Duchene, 2015; Burrell, Ives & Unwin, 2017; Chao et al., 2017). A study by Chao et al. (2017) found that adjusting expectations was a coping mechanism for many parents and that it often led to a new sense of hope and vision for the future. Chao et al. (2017) further found that by adjusting expectations and focusing more on the child's capabilities, parents could increase their ability to cope with stressors. This increase in ability to cope bears a resemblance to Fletcher and Sarkar's (2013) definition of resilience, specifically the ability to cope amidst life's difficulties. It can therefore be concluded that the respondents in Chao et al.'s (2017) study, as well as the respondents in this study, displayed a level of resilience as seen by adjusting their expectations of their children in order to cope.

Acceptance of the child with the diagnosis
Most respondents spoke about the importance of getting to a place of acceptance of the child with their diagnosis as a form of coping.

Whether he has the diagnosis or not... no matter how much he's progressed... I have accepted it from the beginning... But I think if you're in denial, it's harder because how can you help the child if you don't believe it? ... If you accept it and talk about it, it's easier to manage. (Respondent 3, Female, 31)

The biggest thing is you've got to embrace your child and accept them, 100%. You can't be sad for the person who you think they should have been or the person who's stuck inside. That person isn't there. (Respondent 10, Female, 48)

I'm in a space where autism is not a life sentence at all... I just see my son as beautiful and talented and intelligent and unique, and autism is just part of who he is right now. And we totally embrace it... I think loving and accepting them and celebrating them for who they are today is the most important. Yes, you can invest in therapy and have dreams and goals for them... But I think it needs to be balanced with [the message that you] deserve love and you're beautiful and you're amazing and we can celebrate you for who you are right now without having to change you... Like any child, they want affection and affirmation and acceptance. So that's what makes autism much easier for me. (Respondent 14, Female, 43)

Most respondents coped by accepting their child with their diagnosis, as can be seen in some of the examples above. This finding echoed Burrell, Ives and Unwin (2017), as well as Selman et al. (2017), who found that the acceptance of one's child with their ASD diagnosis could be a form of coping for parents.

Previous research has found various ways in which parents have come to a place of accepting their child's ASD diagnosis. Berhane (2016) found that parents, through increasing their knowledge on ASD, were able to accept their child with their diagnosis. Additionally, both Tadesse (2014) and Selman et al. (2017) found that parents reframed ASD in their attempt to accept their child's diagnosis. While respondents in this study were not specifically asked how they came to accept their child with their diagnosis, respondents mentioned both increasing their knowledge of, and reframing, ASD in their responses to other questions within the interview. For example, most respondents spoke about increasing their knowledge on ASD as a form of coping, which will be explored in a subcategory below. Respondents also spoke about adjusting their future expectations, hopes, and dreams for their child, which could be a form of reframing ASD. DePape and Lindsay (2015) also found that parents might come to accept their child with their ASD by making ASD a normal part of family life (DePape and Lindsay, 2015).

As a result of the finding that most parents in this study coped by accepting their child with their diagnosis, one could conclude that acceptance is one of the respondents' *internal protective factors*. As stated in resiliency theory, protective factors increase a person's ability to face and overcome difficulties (Greene, Galambos & Lee, 2004). Previous research agrees that acceptance could increase a parent's resilience, as Selman et al. (2017) found that those who find acceptance are better able to cope when stigmatised. Burrell, Ives and Unwin (2017) also found that acceptance could lead to a better ability to cope with others' negative responses towards their child's diagnosis. It can therefore be concluded that the respondents in this study who found acceptance of their child with their diagnosis were better able to cope with other difficulties as a result.

4.4.2.1.3. Personal growth of the parent
Most respondents shared that caring for a child living with ASD has led to personal growth. The most common aspects of personal growth reported, were those of growing in patience and empathy.

I'm much, much, much more patient... I've also become that much more empathetic, so because [my child] can't tell me verbally what he wants or needs, or how he's feeling or if he's in pain, I have to look at all his non-verbal cues... I think, for me, besides the patience and empathy, just celebrating every moment... Any achievement is a big achievement for us as a family... and just being more loveable. (Respondent 15, Female, 34)

From an intellectual point of view... it definitely teaches you to be resilient and more resourceful. (Respondent 17, Female, 51)

It just changes you as a person, but for the better... I think that you do have a different outlook on life... And you enjoy the little things. You can't wait for the big things... You can grow as a person. It can make you stronger. (Respondent 20, Female, 46)

Personal development was one of the mechanisms that enabled respondents to cope. One of the most common aspects of personal growth in this study was an increase in patience, which was also found in previous studies (Corcoran, Berry & Hill, 2015; DePape & Lindsay, 2015; Duchene, 2015; Berhane, 2016; Burrell, Ives & Unwin, 2017). Other areas of personal growth reported by the respondents in this study included an increase in emotional strength, acceptance of and compassion for others, gratitude, humility, and resilience, and a decrease in selfishness. As in this study, previous studies have found that, through the caring of a child living with ASD, many parents grow in their acceptance of others (Corcoran, Berry & Hill, 2015; DePape & Lindsay, 2015; Berhane, 2016; Burrell, Ives & Unwin, 2017).

Respondents stated that personal growth helped them to cope with caring for their child. Respondents' personal growth could therefore be seen as being *internal protective factors* (Greene, Galambos & Lee, 2004). These internal factors help respondents to face and overcome adversity, leading to an increase in resilience, as described in resiliency theory (Greene, Galambos & Lee, 2004). Personal growth could therefore be seen as a way in which parents could increase their overall resilience.

4.4.2.2. Practical ways of coping

Another category that was found under the theme of coping mechanisms was that parents also sought practical ways of coping with caring for their children living with ASD. Sub-categories that were found included managing their child's difficult behaviours, utilising a blend of interventions for their child, and educating oneself and others on ASD.

4.4.2.2.1. Management of their child's difficult behaviours

Most respondents stated that, in order to cope, they tried to manage their children's difficult behaviours. Respondents often attempted to do this by trying to prevent difficult behaviours before they occurred.

We've obviously set up our home. We've always had a trampoline. I have lots of hammocks in my garden. Sometimes they work. We've got this elasticised sleeping bag thing that [my child] used to lie in... We pop popcorn because there's calming sensation in your jaw... Getting into the bath. But their sensory profiles change. So when [my child] used to calm down getting into the bath, eventually the bath didn't work anymore and we had to keep exploring other ways to calm down... We try to distract her. Try to hold her. She likes to be tickled. We tickle her face. Brush her hair. Lie on the bed with her... It's better to just be home... [We] totally avoid the shops... But it's the preparation. We can't just decide while we're driving home, let's quickly stop at [the shop] and get some stuff. It doesn't work like that... They often have insomnia. And we've learned to deal with it... She listens to her music really softly and then I try give her [medication] to go back to sleep. (Respondent 9, Female, 46)

There are times when we need to sit down and someone can't watch him all the time and then we lock the bedroom and bathroom doors... One of the things we were taught... was to be your child's narrator. So we would always tell him what's going to be happening next... [When he's spitting water in public] we try to give him something else... So we would try giving him an alternative to keep him busy that's more socially appropriate... We try to give him limits... I guess inside the home it's a bit easier, because you just don't buy ornaments and you just keep everything high up. And you don't buy expensive furniture and things like that... We always have to have one eye on [him]... There are just certain places we just don't go. (Respondent 14, Female, 43)

Most respondents attempted to cope by managing their children's difficult behaviours, particularly through preventative methods. This finding was consistent with the findings of both Duchene (2015) and Berhane (2016), who found that prevention was a key way that parents attempted to cope with their children's difficult behaviours. Both Duchene (2015) and Berhane (2016) found that the main way that parents attempted to prevent their children's difficult behaviours was through providing and implementing schedules and routine for their children. However, the findings of this study were a lot more varied, and there was a plethora of ways in which the respondents reported attempting to prevent their children's difficult behaviours. It could therefore be concluded that, while the findings of this study was in keeping with the results of other studies that parents primarily attempted to manage their children's behaviours through the use of prevention, the ways in which this was done differed between respondents.

4.4.2.2.2. Utilisation of a blend of interventions from HCPs and other professionals
All respondents used a blend of interventions from HCPs and other professionals for their children. The most common interventions were provided by Occupational and Speech Therapists. Examples of other interventions that were utilised by HCPs included using various communication systems and psychiatric medications.

So when he was five... they introduced this [communication] system... That was a lifesaver for us... He continued with his speech [therapy]... and then the words started coming and slowly but surely he... just started speaking... So he's really come a long way... So from the diagnosis we went onto [medication]... and then we started the behavioural management with him. So a lot of it was behavioural teaching and that helped us a lot. It was a lot of work...But we were given homework... and I could get the just of what needed to be done... So he was sort of getting continuous therapy at home. (Respondent 5, Female, 40)

He's been with this speech therapist since he was two and a half... he had [Occupational Therapy] at that school as well. So maybe that's when I saw the psychiatrist... The [medication] has definitely been a god-sent in that the meltdowns are less... And [we have] the most wonderful speech therapist... [My child] has a bond with her and he is visibly calmer after he's seen her. I think it's his safe place. (Respondent 8, Female, 44)

In this study, it was found that all respondents utilised a blend of interventions for their children. This finding confirmed Eyal et al.'s (2010) research, which found that, because ASD exists on a spectrum, many different intervention options are needed. Due to the spectrum, the National Institute of Mental Health USA (2018) found that the blend of interventions needed varies from person-to-person. It could therefore be concluded that respondents within this study utilise a range of different interventions that are specific to their child's needs.

Utilising a blend of interventions from HCPs and other professionals seemed to be an *external protective factor* for respondents, leading to an increase in resilience and therefore the ability to cope, as defined in Greene, Galambos and Lee's (2004) resiliency theory. It could therefore be said that utilising a blend of interventions could provide respondents with the increased ability to cope with adversity. This concurs with research by Corcoran, Berry and Hill (2015), who found that providing appropriate intervention strategies for children prevented difficult behaviours and enabled parents to cope as a result.

4.4.2.2.3. Educating themselves on ASD

Most respondents reported that one of the ways they coped was by educating themselves on ASD. This included using search engines on the Internet, reading books and online blogs, and attending workshops and courses. In this study, when asked what respondents would recommend to other parents, the majority of them said to educate themselves on ASD.

You realise that the more information you've got and the knowledge and understanding you've got certainly helps you in that process... You've got a lot of learning to do... And I read a lot of blogs about autism... Brilliant autistic people are now blogging. A lot of them have written books. It's fascinating to see the world from their perspective. I think it helps you have a lot of insight into your own child. (Respondent 10, Female, 48)

I also went into a major mission of just researching as much as I possibly could... To try and be a little bit positive, I looked at a lot of success stories on people with autism and what they have been able to achieve in their lives. Since then, we've gone on many courses to try and help him... Do the reading. Understand your child. Understand what his behaviours are and that he doesn't want to be naughty. He doesn't want to act out and throw tantrums and do these things. (Respondent 15, Female, 34)

Most respondents went through the effort of educating themselves on ASD in an attempt to cope. This was in line with previous studies that found that educating oneself was a common coping mechanism used by parents post-diagnosis (Kuhaneck et al., 2010; Marshall & Long, 2010; Berhane, 2016; Burrell, Ives & Unwin, 2017; Selman et al., 2017). Furthermore, a finding by Berhane (2016) stated that some parents increased their knowledge of ASD by speaking to fellow parents who had children living with ASD. Looking to other parents as a way of increasing knowledge may be true for this study as many respondents mentioned reading blogs by, and interacting on social media with, other parents as necessary forms of self-education. From the above findings, it could be concluded that educating oneself was an especially effective form of coping for respondents, as it was also the recommendation that most respondents made to other parents caring for children living with ASD.

Most respondents mentioned that they attempted to educate others as a form of coping with some of the impacts of caring for a child living with ASD. Respondents frequently attempted to educate members of the public, their community, and their family. The most common way of educating others was through the use of verbal communication.

Some people, when you go to the shop or some public place, they will always stare at this child and it's like we're aliens and we're from another planet. But I will go to them and say, "Listen, he's autistic. That's the way he is and that's why he's doing this." (Respondent 2, Female, 50)

But now what I often do in the shops... [is] they'd give me a disgusting look and the first thing I'd say is that my child struggles to communicate verbally, so he's shouting because he doesn't know how to say the words. And then people go, "Oh, okay."... As long as they understand what's going on, I actually don't care. (Respondent 11, Female, 31)

When he was 4 [years old] we had a little card made at the school that says this child has got autism and can't stand in queues for long and this is how it might manifest... If he was a bit disruptive where I could see people were going to be nasty then I'd just show the card and not say anything. I still have that as a backup, but now because I'm comfortable I try to use it as a teaching moment... [He] would [also] wear one of those [T-shirts] that says, "I'm not naughty, I'm autistic," and it explains the traits on the back... We did a drive last year April where we had those posters and little fliers... I try to speak about it openly with friends and family... My first April autism awareness, I changed my [social media] profile to something that teaches them about autism or teaches them how autism parents feel. (Respondent 14, Female, 43)

The finding that respondents attempted to educate others on ASD as a form of coping was one that has also been found in various other studies (Kuhaneck et al., 2010; Marshall & Long, 2010; Neely-Barnes et al., 2011; Lutz, Patterson & Klein, 2012). Respondents seemed to educate others as a way of coping with the perceived judgement that they experienced from them, as well as others' seeming ignorance regarding ASD. These reasons were also found in previous research that was conducted by Marshall and Long

(2010). The people who respondents spent time educating the most were people who they did not know and who came into contact with their children in public spaces. Respondents also spent time educating family members, which was also found in a study by Lutz, Patterson and Klein (2012).

4.4.3. Support mechanisms

Two categories emerged in relation to the third objective of the study, which was to determine what support mechanisms parents of children living with ASD need to cope effectively. These consisted of support from family and from fellow parents also caring for children living with ASD.

4.4.3.1. Support from family

Most respondents said that they received support from their families, which often included support from respondents' partners, siblings and parents. Respondents reported feeling supported by their family's display of empathy and understanding towards the realities of caring for a child living with ASD, their acceptance towards the child, and their practical help.

> *Our family... were very supportive from the beginning and tried to help as much as they could. I could go to my mother and she would help me... I could call [my sisters] and they would help me... I feel that my husband and myself were definitely on the same page from the beginning. I think it would have been harder if the one wanted to do something and the other one didn't. But both of us had that same drive. Both of us were always on Google or reading books or trying to find out new stuff... My husband is extremely involved. (Respondent 3, Female, 31)*

> *We actually have two more special needs kids in the [extended] family. Both are autistic as well. So [the extended family has] been completely accepting. We're a tribe of weirdos and we're all happy with that... I wouldn't be able to do this on my own. My husband didn't give up on me, my friends didn't give up on me, [and] my family didn't give up on me. They've given me the strength to become strong again. (Respondent 11, Female, 31)*

Familial support was one of the primary ways in which respondents gained support. This finding is consistent with the findings of both Corcoran, Berry and Hill (2015) and Hall and

Graff (2010), who found that parents often gained support from family members. Previous research from Hartley, DaWalt and Schultz (2017) found that many parents gained support from their spouses and that this support helped them to cope. Furthermore, Corcoran, Berry and Hill (2015) found that for those parents who have spouses, spousal support was the biggest form of support received. This was the case for the majority of respondents within this study as they reported that support from their respective life partners helped them to cope.

Whilst, in this study, some respondents spoke about needing to educate members of their family, the great majority of respondents still found that they experienced much of their support from family. Blanche et al. (2015) found that extended family members were a form of support for parents, however they were often slow and resistant to accepting the child's diagnosis of ASD, which might explain why respondents still felt the need to educate them. In this study, respondents referred to their mothers and sisters more often than to fathers and brothers when it came to support, which is similar to Blanche et al.'s (2015) finding that the extended familial support that mothers received was mostly from other female family members.

4.4.3.2. Informal support from other parents
Most respondents said that they received support from other parents who also cared for children living with ASD. Respondents shared that support from other parents usually occurred through face-to-face contact, and through social media and messaging groups. Gaining informal support from other parents was also a recommendation that respondents suggested for parents who had just received a diagnosis of ASD for their children.

Other parents are a fantastic way to get assistance... Just finding other mothers who understand what you're going through. Because one thing is certain: no one else gets it like the mother of another autistic child. There's just no doubt about that! So that's also been quite healing and helpful over the years... Also going to friends who also have autistic children and socialising with them is a good idea because then they are really sympathetic. They know what your concerns are. They are very safety conscious... It's really nice because then the kids can play together. We can almost have that feeling of normality that we've just never had... And I think that's the importance of talking to other moms who can then say, "Well yes, our kid was also like that when he was 7 [years old], but now he's 10 and it's so much easier." (Respondent 10, Female, 48)

I'm on a couple of WhatsApp support groups for autism moms, so when days do get bad I reach out and I'm like, "I'm having one of those days where I just want to give up and run away. I hate autism! I hate everything today and what [ASD has] done to [my child]." And it's okay. They give me support and the next day it'll be better... Talking to somebody who gets it. Talking to somebody who understands or who's been through it or is going through it is a huge thing. (Respondent 15, Female, 34)

I started trying to meet parents who also have autistic children. I just went out there to try and find them. And [the parents] helped me a lot... They have a lot of advice because they have been down the road a bit already... Become friends with other autistic people's families because those people are worth gold... And they can give you a lot of advice... That's where I learned the most. (Respondent 19, Female, 48)

The above quotes are examples of the finding that informal support from other parents was a key source of support for respondents. These findings reflected previous studies that reported on how beneficial support from other parents could be (Ammari, Morris & Schoenebeck, 2014; Berhane, 2016; Burrell, Ives & Unwin, 2017).

Respondents were specific about the informal nature of their interactions with other parents. This finding was surprising as it contradicted previous research by Crane et al (2015), who recommended that parents be referred to more formal support groups as they found this was most effective. While respondents did not mention gaining support from formal groups, it could be concluded that formal support groups were either not utilised or not as effective for them, as they were rarely mentioned. Another possibility is that there may not have been many formal groups available to respondents within the South African context, which could have influenced the findings. In this study, it was unclear as to why respondents mentioned informal rather than formal means of connecting with other parents. One reason for the informal nature of support could be due to the flexibility that it gives respondents. This echoes Schaff et al.'s (2011) study, which found that one of the key ways in which parents coped with their child's ASD-related needs was to be flexible within their daily routines. In this study, flexibility could have been beneficial due to the number of stressors that respondents experienced in caring for a child living with ASD. Flexibility would therefore give respondents the ability to connect with other parents in whatever way suited them and at a time that was most convenient for them. Within this study, the ability to be flexible might have also increased respondents' resilience, especially taking into consideration Greef and Van Der Walt's (2010) finding that flexibility was a key aspect of resiliency for the respondents in their study.

Social media was mentioned multiple times by respondents with regard to gaining informal support from other parents. Social media included the use of WhatsApp and Facebook. This study did not address the reasons why parents used social media in their efforts to gain support, however, its use could be due to the informal nature of social media, as mentioned above. Ammari, Morris and Schoenebeck (2014) found that many people have the perception that there is less judgement from others on social media platforms as opposed to face-to-face, and that it is a safer space for people to seek support as a result. It is possible that the perception of there being less judgment within the social media space could be a reason why respondents within this study utilised these platforms.

4.5. Conclusion

In conclusion, this chapter provided a demographic profile of the respondents, as well as a framework of analysis, which provided a format in which to present the findings of the study. The themes of stressors, coping mechanisms and support mechanisms were investigated. Stressors revolved around the child's ASD symptoms, the practicalities of caring for a child living with ASD, and parents' own emotions, whilst coping mechanisms were either of a psychological or practical nature. Support mechanisms that were found consisted of support from family members and from other parents who care for a child living with ASD.

5.1. Introduction

This chapter begins by providing the conclusions for each of the three objectives of this study. Thereafter, recommendations are made to HCPs and organisations working in the field, as well as to parents, and recommendations for further research are given.

5.2. Conclusions

The conclusions of this study will be presented under each of the three objectives. The objectives were to explore the stressors faced by parents of children living with ASD, to explore the coping strategies that parents use in caring for children living with ASD, and to determine what support mechanisms parents of children living with ASD need to cope effectively.

5.2.1. Objective 1: To explore the stressors faced by parents of children living with ASD

Numerous stressors are prevalent in caring for a child living with ASD, according to the respondents of this study. Stressors relate to the child's ASD symptoms, the stressors related to the practicalities of caring for the child, and the stressors experienced as a result of the parents' own emotions.

Managing their child's ASD-related behaviours was overwhelmingly experienced as a stressor within this study, with every single respondent highlighting their experience of this. The experience of managing their children's behaviours was exacerbated for many of the parents in this study by their attempts to prevent these difficult behaviours from occurring. So as to prevent embarrassment, parents seemed especially concerned about managing these behaviours when they occurred in public. Whilst stressors related to managing behaviours may be prevalent in parenting children in general, respondents highlighted the ASD-specific nature of their child's behaviours. This included unpredictability and rigidity, along with behaviours that would be deemed as socially inappropriate.

The child's difficult to manage, ASD-related behaviours that respondents mentioned above often led to an increase in respondents' anxiety levels, especially as parents needed to remain vigilant at all times when with their child, so as to ensure their child's safety. This meant that respondents' anxiety levels were found to be particularly high, and that these high anxiety levels were found to be a stressor for respondents as a result.

Respondents also spoke about the difficulties related to their struggle to communicate with their child. Many respondents mentioned the frustration that their child experienced due to being unable to effectively communicate their needs, often leading to meltdowns and an increase in adverse behaviours. Respondents found that the difficulty to communicate, and the resulting frustration from their child, was a stressor.

Respondents also shared the stressors that they experienced due to the practicalities related to caring for their child, the most frustrating of which was the long time that it took to receive a diagnosis for their child based on needing to consult multiple HCPs. This often included needing to rule out various other diagnoses before their child could receive a confirmed diagnosis of ASD. Once parents received an official diagnosis of ASD for their child, they were then faced with the additional stressor of the high costs related to providing their child with necessary care and interventions. This was compounded by the difficulty that respondents experienced in finding an affordable and appropriate school for their child, where they felt that their child's special needs were catered for. As a result of this stressor, many respondents moved their child between schools, hoping to find one that they felt suited their child. While some parents had eventually found an appropriate school that they could afford, others were still on this journey.

The respondents' own emotions related to some of the aforementioned stressors and were experienced as stressors in and of themselves. Many parents experienced negative emotions, including grief and loss, when they finally received a diagnosis of ASD for their child. The loss of the preconceived notions that they had of their child before they received the diagnosis of ASD was experienced by many respondents, as was anxiety about their child's future as a result. Future concerns centred on how the child would cope if they were to lose their parents, as well as how they would remain socially connected and would be able to provide for themselves and become independent. Another emotion that many respondents found to be a stressor in their lives was the hurt that they felt as a result of other people not understanding ASD and judging them and their child as a result, which seemed to lead to respondents trying to educate other people on ASD to mitigate this.

From the above conclusions, it was clear that respondents experienced a multitude of stressors in caring for a child living with ASD. This, therefore, proved challenging for respondents and presented them with various difficulties that they needed to attempt to cope with. These stressors were found to be over and above the usual stressors that respondents faced regarding the usual care required for a child, regardless of whether they have a diagnosis.

5.2.2. Objective 2: To explore the coping strategies that parents use in caring for children living with ASD

Respondents within this study displayed resilience and coped with the above-mentioned stressors through a variety of coping strategies, which were either psychological or practical in nature.

One of the key psychological coping strategies that respondents utilised was adjusting their expectations and hopes for their child's future, which seemed to create a sense of renewed hope and an alternate vision for respondents for their child. Coupled with this, was reaching acceptance for their child with their diagnosis. Acceptance led to respondents being able to embrace their child. It also enabled them to move on from mourning their preconceived notions of what their child would be like before receiving the diagnosis. Acceptance could have been a result of respondents' attempts to increase in their understanding of ASD, as well as reframing it for themselves. Along with acceptance, many respondents found that through their journey of caring for their child, they increased in their ability to display patience, acceptance and empathy towards others, which further enabled them to cope with the stressors that they faced.

Along with the psychological coping strategies that respondents utilised to cope, they also made use of various practical coping strategies, one of which was the management of their child's difficult ASD-related behaviours. Managing their child's difficult behaviours was often done through the use of prevention, as mentioned above, however, the way in which respondents attempted to prevent these behaviours varied greatly, and no one strategy was found to be more common than others. Aside from the management and prevention of behaviours, respondents attempted to educate both themselves and others on ASD as a form of coping. Most respondents recommended that other parents educate themselves as a form of coping, especially to gather relevant information. When speaking about educating others, most respondents spoke about using verbal means to educate others, which ranged from complete strangers in public places to close family members. A heightened understanding of ASD by others was also found to increase the support that respondents received, especially when these people had a close relationship with respondents.

In keeping with the topic of practical coping strategies that respondents employed, all respondents mentioned utilising a blend of interventions from HCPs and other professionals for their children. The blend of interventions used varied for each child based on their specific presentation, although this often included the use of Occupational Therapists, Speech Therapists, and professionals who incorporated communication systems and psychiatric medications. However, as per the stressors discussed previously, interventions were found to be costly for parents, and so these same interventions that enabled respondents to cope seemed to add to their number of stressors as well. Therefore, the cost of these same interventions might have also led to an increase in financial stress for respondents.

5.2.3. Objective 3: To determine what support mechanisms parents of children living with ASD need to cope effectively

Drawing from the sentiments in this study, it can be concluded that respondents utilised two main support mechanisms that assisted them in coping with caring for a child living with ASD. The most prevalent form of support that respondents mentioned was from their families, especially when family members displayed empathy towards them, understood the stressors that they were facing, and assisted them on a practical level. This was especially true for those respondents who had a life partner. Notably, even while respondents were still in the process of educating family members who did not fully understand ASD, these same family members gave most of the respondents support.

Other parents who cared for a child living with ASD were found to be a support to respondents, especially when their support was informal and allowed respondents to remain flexible within their daily routines. Many of the interactions that respondents had with other parents took place over social media platforms, such as WhatsApp and

Facebook, which could have been the case due to their being less perceived intimidation and judgement over social media than in face-to-face interactions. Accessing informal support from other parents was another recommendation that respondents gave to other parents caring for a child with ASD, which highlights how beneficial respondents found these interactions to be.

5.3. Recommendations

Various recommendations have been made based on the findings of this study. The recommendations consist of those made: to HCPs and other professionals working within the field of ASD, to social work practice, to organisations working within the field of ASD, to parents, and for future research.

5.3.1. Recommendations to HCPs and other professionals working within the field of ASD

- HCPs and other professionals working within the field of ASD are well positioned to provide education and referral information to parents with regard to ASD. This is especially true when parents first receive an official diagnosis for their child. HCPs who diagnose children with ASD are therefore especially ideally situated to provide education to parents when diagnosis occurs. This could be beneficial as respondents within this study found education to be a key coping mechanism in caring for a child living with ASD. It is recommended that HCPs and other professionals therefore increase their own knowledge of ASD and related services and interventions, so that they can pass this information on to parents during their contact time with them.

- Furthermore, HCP's and other professionals can offer education on the management of the child's symptoms. This can include providing information and training on interventions that develop the child's communication skills. This could be especially beneficial, as it may lower frustration and stress levels in parents. It is also recommended that HCPs and organisations within the field increase their knowledge as to how parents can manage and prevent their child's difficult behaviours, seeing as this was a key coping mechanism for respondents in this study.

- HCPs and other professionals working within the field of ASD are also often privy to parents' emotional responses, especially once parents receive an official diagnosis of ASD for their child. It is recommended that HCPs and other professionals normalise and allow parents to mourn the loss of the child they thought they had prior to obtaining their child's diagnosis, and to support parents in such a way that parents are able to accept their child with their diagnosis. HCPs and other professionals should refer parents for counselling and link them to support groups. These could allow parents to process and normalise their feelings of loss, as well as to find strategies to cope with the array of stressors that they might face as a result of caring for a child living with ASD, as was found in this study.

- HCPs and other professionals working within the field of ASD are ideally positioned to be able to link parents to appropriate services and schooling. It is recommended that HCPs and other professionals are aware of the service providers and schooling available in their area, as well as in surrounding areas. HCPs and other professionals could make contact with these organisations so that they know what is offered and can provide specialised referrals to parents through the networking they have done.

- HCPs and other professionals working within the field of ASD are also in the unique position where they meet multiple parents caring for a child living with ASD. It is recommended that HCPs and other professionals link parents with one another in such a way that they can be introduced and then make their own connections in more informal ways going forward. This would allow parents to learn from one another and to support each other in a manner and time that suits them.

5.3.2. Recommendations for social work practice

Although social workers are included in the aforementioned recommendations for *HCPs and other professionals working within the field of ASD*, the following additional recommendations can be made specifically for social work practice.

- One of the underpinnings of social work practice is to utilise a strengths-based approach when working with clients. Within this study, the importance of identifying strengths in order to build resilience in parents caring for a child living with ASD has been highlighted. It is therefore recommended that social workers assist parents caring for a child with ASD to identify and tap into their strengths so as to increase their, and their families', levels of resilience.

- Social workers are in the unique position where they could utilise their skills to advocate for parents caring for a child living with ASD, especially with regard to adding to and ensuring the implementation of policy and legislation that could assist these parents in caring for their children, as well as to advocate for and connect parents to social services, such as financial grants.

- Social workers work from a holistic, systems-based approach, and have a broad skills set. It is therefore recommended that, when necessary and where possible, social workers assist in filling in the gaps where other HCPs and professionals working within the field of ASD are unable to meet the needs of parents caring for a child living with ASD.

5.3.3. Recommendations to organisations working within the field of ASD

- Many organisations working within the field of ASD offer access to various services and interventions for children living with ASD. As respondents in this study noted the high cost of care and interventions available for their children, it is recommended that organisations come up with ways in which they can make their services more affordable to those who are unable to afford them. This could be done through strategies such as providing a sliding scale in which those who earn less money pay a decreased fee for services, or by implementing fundraising initiatives so that money raised can assist those who are unable to afford their services.

- Organisations working within the field may also have opportunities to share their knowledge of ASD with parents who care for a child living with ASD, as well as with greater society. It is recommended that organisations work to come up with ways in which they can make information on ASD more widely and easily accessible. This could include the provision of hardcopy resources, workshops, and resources online. Online resources could be provided through the use of organisations' websites and social media platforms, such as Facebook, so that parents and others are able to access information easily from wherever it is they might find themselves.

5.3.4. Recommendations to parents

- Education was one of the key coping strategies that respondents used in this study. It is recommended that parents educate themselves on ASD, for example through the resources provided by various organisations, or by speaking to other parents who care for a child living with ASD, researching ASD online, or reading ASD-related books.

- It is also recommended that parents find ways to educate others on ASD. This could be attempted by: providing resources for others, for example by handing out fliers and sharing helpful links to information via social media; having informative conversations with others; and sharing their ASD-related experiences. The hope would be that educating others would increase other people's knowledge on ASD, thereby increasing support for parents caring for children living with ASD, and thereby decreasing stigmatisation.

- Parents could benefit from finding ways to improve their communication with their child, especially due to the stressors that seem to exist when there is the struggle to communicate with one another. It is therefore recommended that parents find additional, alternate forms of communicating with their child aside from verbal conversation, and that they utilise a blend of interventions that target their child's ability to communicate more effectively.

- As seen in this study, respondents experience various negative emotions as a result of caring for a child living with ASD, particularly when their child received an official diagnosis. It could, therefore, be helpful for parents to allow themselves a period of time to mourn once their child has received a diagnosis of ASD, and to, thereafter, work towards accepting their child with their diagnosis. Parents could also spend time with other parents caring for a child living with ASD and normalise the emotions that other parents have experienced, thereby potentially giving other parents the permission to feel whatever emotion it is that they feel. It is recommended that parents who need assistance in processing their difficult emotions speak to other parents with a child living with ASD, supportive family or friends, or go for counselling, so that they are able to talk through their feelings and experiences.

- Respondents in this study primarily received their support from family members, life partners, and other parents caring for a child living with ASD. Due to the importance of support, it is recommended that parents reach out to empathetic friends and family when support is needed, and that they refrain from isolating themselves. It is also recommended that parents spend time getting to know other parents who have a child living with ASD, and to share some of their stressors and coping mechanisms with other parents so that they are able to learn from one another.

- When looking to the future, parents could benefit from planning potential alternate care and financial arrangements for their child, in case this is needed. This is recommended so as to decrease potential feelings of anxiety and fear related to their child's future, especially with regard to their child's future independence and financial stability.

5.3.5. Recommendations for future research

- A gap was found in previous research with regard to the prevalence of ASD within South Africa, as previous studies have either focused on global prevalence or prevalence within the USA. It is therefore recommended that the prevalence of ASD within South Africa be researched.
- In this study, it was unclear as to the different socioeconomic statuses of respondents, however, it seemed that most respondents could have fallen within a higher economic bracket, especially due to the resources that they mentioned utilising. It is therefore recommended that future research look at the differences between parents who come from different socioeconomic backgrounds within South Africa, as this would particularly influence the resources available to parents.
- Respondents in this study came from major cities within South Africa and did not live in outlying areas. Future research on parents living in outlying areas is recommended, especially as the findings could lead to differences in resources and support structures available, depending on where the outlying area is situated within South Africa.
- The ease of accessibility to various intervention strategies and appropriate schooling within South Africa was not explored in-depth within this study. Resultantly, this could be an aspect for future research, as, within the literature review, it was found that gaining access could be a challenge for respondents.
- This study was open to both mothers and fathers caring for a child living with ASD in South Africa. However, only mothers volunteered to take part. It is recommended that future researchers explore the stressors, coping mechanisms and support structures of fathers. This may uncover important differences between the experiences of mothers and fathers in caring for a child living with ASD.
- One of the key coping strategies that respondents mentioned was accepting their child with their diagnosis. However, this study did not fully explore how respondents came to acceptance. Future research could therefore explore the ways in which respondents could learn to accept their child with their diagnosis, thereby benefitting

other parents by enabling them to more readily accept their child with their diagnosis too.

5.4. Conclusion

To conclude, the paper began by introducing the study. This included the statement of the problem, rationale of the research, research topic, main research questions and objectives, concept clarification, and ethical considerations. The paper then provided a review of the literature, including key theoretical models and relevant policy and legislation. The methodology of the research was then addressed, including: the research design; sampling; data collection, analysis and verification; reflexivity; and limitations. Thereafter, the findings were presented. This included the demographic profile of respondents, framework of analysis, and presentation of findings with regard to stressors faced by parents, as well as coping and support mechanisms available. Conclusions to the three research objectives were then provided, followed by recommendations made to HCPs, social work practice, organisations and parents, and for future research.

References

American Psychiatric Association. 2013. *Diagnostic and statistical manual of mental disorders*. 5th ed. Washington DC: American Psychiatric Publishing.

Ammari, T., Morris, M.R. & Schoenebeck, S.Y. 2014. Accessing social support and overcoming judgment on social media among parents of children with special needs. In *Eighth International AAAI Conference on Weblogs and Social Media*. 22–31.

Babbie, E. & Mouton, J. 2001. *The practice of social research*. SA ed. Cape Town: Oxford University Press.

Baxter, A.J., Brugha, T.S., Erskine, H.E., Scheurer, R.W., Vos, T. & Scott, J.G. 2015. The epidemiology and global burden of autism spectrum disorders. *Psychological Medicine*. 45:601–613.

Berhane, H. 2016. *Reactions, challenges and coping mechanisms of mothers raising children with autism spectrum disorder (ASD): the case of Addis Ababa City*. MA. book. Addis Ababa University.

Blanche, E.I., Diaz, J., Barretto, T. & Cermak, S.A. 2015. Caregiving experiences of Latino families with children with autism spectrum disorder. *American Journal of Occupational Therapy*. 69(5):1–11.

Breen, A., Swartz, L., Flisher, A.J., Joska, J.A., Corrigall, J., Plaatjies, L. & McDonald, D.A. 2007. Experience of mental disorders in the context of basic service reforms: the impact on caregiving environments in South Africa. *International Journal of Environmental Health Research*. 17(5):327–334.

Burrell, A., Ives, J. & Unwin, G. 2017. The experiences of fathers who have offspring with autism spectrum disorder. *Journal of Autism and Developmental Disorders*. 47(4):1135–1147.

Centers for Disease Control and Prevention. 2014a. *Community report on autism*. Available: http://www.cdc.gov/ncbddd/autism/states/comm_report_autism_2014.pdf [2017, May 03].

Centers for Disease Control and Prevention. 2014b. Prevalence of autism spectrum disorder among children aged 8 years - Autism and Developmental Disabilities Monitoring Network, 11 sites, United States, 2010. *Surveillance Summaries*. 63(2):1–21. Available: http://www.ncbi.nlm.nih.gov/pubmed/24670961 [2017, May 06].

Centers for Disease Control and Prevention. 2018. Prevalence of autism spectrum
disorder among children aged 8 years - Autism and Developmental Disabilities
Monitoring Network, 11 Sites, United States, 2014. *Surveillance Summaries*.
67(6):1–23. Available https://www.cdc.gov/mmwr/volumes/67/ss/ss6706a1.htm
[2019, December 02].

Chambers, N., Wetherby, A., Stronach, S., Njongwe, N., Kauchali, S. & Grinker, R. 2016.
Early detection of autism spectrum disorder in young isiZulu-speaking children in
South Africa. *Autism*: 1-9.

Chao, K., Chang, H., Chin, W., Li, H. & Chen, S. 2017. How Taiwanese parents of children
with autism spectrum disorder experience the process of obtaining a diagnosis: a
descriptive phenomenological analysis. *Autism*. 1–13.

Children's Act, No. 38 of 2005. 2006. Available:
http://www.refworld.org/docid/46b82aa62.html [2017, May 08].

Children's Act, No. 38 of 2005, as amended. 2010. Available:
http://www.ci.uct.ac.za/sites/default/files/image_tool/images/367/Law_reform/Childr
en_Act_guides/consolidated_childrens_act_1april2010.pdf [2020, January 12].

Children's Amendment Bill, No. 244. 2019. Available:
https://www.justice.gov.za/legislation/notices/2019/20190225-gg42248gon244-
ChildrensActAmendment.pdf [2020, January 12].

Chirwa, L. 2012. *The experiences of mothers caring for their school-going children with
physical or mental disabilities in low-income communities: an ecological
perspective*. MA. book. Stellenbosch University.

Corcoran, J., Berry, A. & Hill, S. 2015. The lived experience of US parents of children with
autism spectrum disorders: a systematic review and meta-synthesis. *Journal of
Intellectual Disabilities*. 19(4):356–366.

Crane, L., Chester, J., Goddard, L., Henry, L. & Hill, E. 2015. Experiences of autism
diagnosis: a survey of over 1000 parents in the United Kingdom. *Autism*. 20(2):153–
162.

Creswell, J. 2014. *Research design: qualitative, quantitative and mixed methods
approaches*. 4th ed. California: Sage Publications.

Deakin, H., & Wakefield, K. 2014. Skype interviewing: reflections of two PhD researchers.
Qualitative Research, 14(5):603-616.

DePape, A. & Lindsay, S. 2015. Parents' experiences of caring for a child with autism
spectrum disorder. *Qualitative Health Research*. 25(4):569–583.

Department of Social Development. 2013. *Help for children with autism. 13 May.* Available: http://www.dsd.gov.za/index.php?option=com_content&task=view&id=487&Itemid= 82 [2017, November 23].

Department of Social Development. 2015. *National integrated early childhood development policy. 9 December.* Available: https://www.gov.za/sites/www.gov.za/files/National Integrated ECD Policy (web Version - Final) 01 08 2016a.pdf [2017, November 23].

De Vos, A., Strydom, H. & Delport, C. 2011. *Research at grass roots: for the social sciences and human service professions.* 4th ed. Pretoria: Van Schaik Publishers.

Donvan, J. & Zucker, C. 2016. *In a different key: the story of autism.* London: Allen Lane.

Duchene, M. 2015. *Maternal experiences of parenting children with autism spectrum disorder: a qualitative analysis.* Ph.D. book. University of Maryland.

Eyal, G., Hart, B., Onculer, E., Oren, N. & Rossi, N. 2010. *The autism matrix: the social origins of the autism epidemic.* Cambridge: Polity Press.

Farooq, M.B. & De Villiers, C. 2017. Telephonic qualitative research interviews, when to consider them and how to do them. *Meditari Accountancy Research.* 25(2):291–316.

Fletcher, D. & Sarkar, M. 2013. Psychological resilience: a review and critique of definitions, concepts, and theory. *European Psychologist.* 18(1):12–23.

Folkman, S. & Lazarus, R. 1980. An analysis of coping in a middle-aged community sample. *Journal of Health and Social Behavior.* 21(3):219–239.

Greeff, A. & Van Der Walt, K. 2010. Resilience in families with an autistic child. *Education and Training in Autism and Developmental Disabilities,* 45(3):347–355.

Greene, R., Galambos, C. & Lee, Y. 2004. Resilience theory: theoretical and professional conceptualizations. *Journal of Human Behavior in the Social Environment.* 8(4):75–91.

Hall, H.R. & Graff, J.C. 2010. Parenting challenges in families of children with autism: a pilot study. *Issues in Comprehensive Pediatric Nursing.* 33:187–204.

Hartley, S., Papp, L., Blumenstock, S., Floyd, F. & Goetz, G. 2016. The effect of daily challenges in children with autism on parents' couple problem-solving interactions. *Journal of Family Psychology.* 30(6):732–742.

Hartley, S., DaWalt, L. & Schultz, H. 2017. Daily couple experiences and parent affect in families of children with versus without autism. *Journal of Autism and Developmental Disorders.* 1–14.

Higashida, N. 2017. *Fall down 7 times get up 8: a young man's voice from the silence of autism*. London: Sceptre Books.

Hurlbutt, K. 2011. Experiences of parents who homeschool their children with autism spectrum disorders. *Focus on Autism and Other Developmental Disabilities*. 26(4):239–249.

Iacono, V., Symonds, P & Brown, H. 2016. Skype as a tool for qualitative research interviews. *Sociological Research Online*, 21(2):1-15.

Irvine, A., Drew, P. & Sainsbury, R. 2013. "Am I not answering your questions properly?" Clarification, adequacy and responsiveness in semi-structured telephone and face-to-face interviews. *Qualitative Research*. 13(1):87–106.

Johansson, S. 2016. Parents negotiating change: a middle-class lens on schooling of children with autism in urban India. *Contemporary Education Dialogue*. 13(1):93–120.

Kavaliotis, P. 2017. Resilience of parents with a child with autism spectrum disorders and factors for its potential enhancement: family income and educational level. *Journal of Educational and Developmental Psychology*. 7(1):188–199.

Kuhaneck, H.M., Burroughs, T., Wright, J., Lemanczyk, T. & Darragh, A.R. 2010. A qualitative study of coping in mothers of children with an autism spectrum disorder. *Physical & Occupational Therapy in Pediatrics*. 30(4):340–350.

Leech, N. & Onwuegbuzie, A. 2011. Beyond constant comparison qualitative data analysis: using NVivo. *American Psychological Association*. 26(1):70–84.

Lincoln, Y. & Guba, E. 1985. Naturalistic Enquiry. Newbury Park, CA: Sage Publications

Lutz, H.R., Patterson, B.J. & Klein, J. 2012. Coping with autism: a journey toward adaptation. *Journal of Pediatric Nursing*. 27:206–213.

Marciano, S., Drasgow, E. & Carlson, R. 2015. The marital experiences of couples who include a child with autism. *The Family Journal: Counseling and Therapy for Couples and Families*. 23(2):132–140.

Marshall, V. & Long, B.C. 2010. Coping processes as revealed in the stories of mothers of children with autism. *Qualitative Health Research*. 20(1):105–116.

Mboweni, T. 2019. *2019 Budget Speech*. Available: http://www.treasury.gov.za/documents/National%20Budget/2019/speech/speech.pdf [2019, November 06].

McGeer, V. 2010. The thought and talk of individuals with autism: reflections on Ian Hacking. In *Cognitive disability and its challenge to moral philosophy*. E. Feder

Kittay & L. Carlson, Eds. Chichester: Wiley-Blackwell.

Mealer, M. & Jones, J. 2014. Methodological and ethical issues related to qualitative telephone interviews on sensitive topics. *Nurse Researcher.* 21(4):32–37.

Monare, N. 2015. *Exploring the perceived challenges of single mothers with children diagnosed with autism disorder in the junior phase at Vera school.* MSocSc. book. University of Cape Town.

National Institute of Mental Health USA. 2018. *Autism spectrum disorder.* Available: https://www.nimh.nih.gov/health/topics/autism-spectrum-disorders-asd/index.shtml [2019, January 16].

Neely-Barnes, S.L., Hall, H.R., Roberts, R.J. & Graff, J.C. 2011. Parenting a child with an autism spectrum disorder: public perceptions and parental conceptualizations. *Journal of Family Social Work.* 14:208–225.

Numbeo. 2017. *Cost of living in South Africa.* Available: https://www.numbeo.com/cost-of-living/country_result.jsp?country=South+Africa [2017, May 14].

Olatunji, M. 2014. Contemporary homeschooling in the Republic of South Africa: some lessons for other African nations. *Middle Eastern & African Journal of Educational Research.* (9):4–17.

Rubenstein, L., Schelling, N., Wilczynski, S. & Hooks, E. 2015. Lived experiences of parents of gifted students with autism spectrum disorder: the struggle to find appropriate educational experiences. *Gifted Child Quarterly.* 59(4):283–298.

Schaaf, R., Toth-Cohen, S., Johnson, S., Outten, G. & Benevides, T. 2011. The everyday routines of families of children with autism: examining the impact of sensory processing difficulties on the family. *Autism*, 15(2):1-17.

Selman, L., Fox, F., Aabe, N., Turner, K., Rai, D. & Redwood, S. 2017. "You are labelled by your children's disability" – a community-based, participatory study of stigma among Somali parents of children with autism living in the United Kingdom. *Ethnicity and Health.* 1–16.

Seltzer, M.M., Greenberg, J.S., Hong, J., Smith, L.E., Almeida, D.M., Coe, C. & Stawski, R.S. 2010. Maternal cortisol levels and behavior problems in adolescents and adults with ASD. *Journal of Autism and Developmental Disorders.* 40:457–469.

Shawler, P. & Sullivan, M. 2015. Parental stress, discipline strategies, and child behavior problems in families with young children with autism spectrum disorders. *Focus on Autism and Other Developmental Disabilities.* 1–10.

Silverman, C. 2012. *Understanding autism: parents, doctors, and the history of the disorder*. New Jersey: Princeton University Press.

Siman-Tov, A. & Kaniel, S. 2011. Stress and personal resource as predictors of the adjustment of parents to autistic children: a multivariate model. *Journal of Autism and Developmental Disorders*. 41(7):879–890.

Simelane, A. 2015. The role of resilience and socio-economic status in the parenting of children with autism spectrum disorder in South Africa. MA. book. University of the Witwatersrand.

Smith, L.E., Hong, J., Seltzer, M.M., Greenberg, J.S., Almeida, D.M. & Bishop, S.L. 2010. Daily experiences among mothers of adolescents and adults with autism spectrum disorder. *Journal of Autism and Developmental Disorders*. 40:167–178.

Tadesse, A. 2014. *Families living with a child diagnosed with autism: challenges and coping mechanisms*. MA. book. Addis Ababa University.

Tesch, R. 1990. *Qualitative research: analysis types and software tools*. New York: Falmer Press.

Tong, M. 2011. The client-centered integrative strengths-based approach: ending longstanding conflict between social work values and practice. *Canadian Social Science*. 7(2),15-22.

Valicenti-McDermott, M., Lawson, K., Hottinger, K., Seijo, R., Schechtman, M., Shulman, L. & Shinnar, S. 2015. Parental stress in families of children with autism and other developmental disabilities. *Journal of Child Neurology*. 30(13):1728–1735.

Van Biljon, S., Kritzinger, A. & Geertsema, S. 2015. A retrospective case report on demographic changes of learners at a school for children with autism spectrum disorder in the Gauteng province. *South African Journal of Childhood Education*, 5(1):1–26.

Van Breda, A. 2018. A critical review of resilience theory and its relevance for social work. *Social work (Stellenbosch. Online)*. 54(1):1-18.

Van Der Merwe, C. 2012. *Three mothers' experiences of raising a child who has been diagnosed with autistic disorder*. University of Johannesburg. Available: https://ujdigispace.uj.ac.za [May 06, 2017].

Whitmore, K.E. 2016. Respite care and stress among caregivers of children with autism spectrum disorder: an integrative review. *Journal of Pediatric Nursing*. 31:630–652.

World Health Organisation. 2020. *Health workforce: health professions networks*. Available: https://www.who.int/hrh/professionals/en/ [2020, September 13].

Appendices

Appendix A: Informed Consent Form

Research Title: An Exploration into the Stressors and Coping Strategies of Parents Caring for Children Living with Autism Spectrum Disorder

Thank you for agreeing to participate in this study. These questions are part of a study that seeks to understand the stressors and coping strategies of parents caring for children living with Autism Spectrum Disorder. The interviews are being conducted as part of the fulfilment of the researcher's Masters in Social Science in Clinical Social Work at the University of Cape Town. The information that will be published will not provide any information that will identify you, and your information will be kept strictly confidential.

The study is completely voluntary. Even if you give consent to participate, you do not have to answer any questions you do not want to, and you can opt out of the study at any point, without prejudice.

Signing this document indicates that you understand the information provided above and are in agreement with the terms below. By signing this form you are providing consent to take part in this study. Thank you for your participation.

I _______________________________________(name) agree to participate in the research project identified above, which is being conducted by Robyn Baker, in completion of her Masters in Social Science in Clinical Social Work at the University of Cape Town.

1. I have been given sufficient information about this research project. The purpose of my participation as an interviewee in this project has been explained to me and is clear.

2. My participation as an interviewee in this project is voluntary. There is no explicit or implicit coercion whatsoever to participate. I understand that there is no compensation for participating. I have the right not to answer any of the questions. I understand that I have the right to opt out of the research at any point.

3. Participation involves being interviewed by Robyn Baker.

4. The interview will be one-on-one and will last approximately 60 minutes. It will take place in a private setting so as to ensure that the interview is not overheard or disturbed.

5. I allow the researcher to record the session and take notes with the understanding that my identity will remain confidential to anyone other than the researcher herself.

6. I have been given the explicit guarantee that the researcher will not identify me by name in any reports using information obtained from this interview, and that my confidentiality as a participant in this study will remain secure. I am aware that any publications that arise from the research will be within the same confidentiality agreement and that no identifying details will be disclosed.

I have read and understood the points and statements of this form. I have had all my questions answered to my satisfaction, and I voluntarily agree to participate in this study.

_________________________________   _________________________________

Respondent's Signature   Date

_________________________________   _________________________________

Researcher's Signature   Date

For further information, please contact:

Researcher: **Research Supervisor**
Robyn Baker   Cindee Bruyns
robyndej@yahoo.com   cindee.bruyns@uct.ac.za
084 012 6468

Appendix B: Interview Schedule

<u>Research Title: An Exploration into the Stressors and Coping Strategies of Parents Caring for Children Living with Autism Spectrum Disorder</u>

1. Introduction

1.1. Introduce self

1.2. Clarify that this is for Masters' research

1.3. Go over consent form

1.4. Thank respondent for agreeing to participate

1.5. As in consent form, ensure they understand confidentiality of recording and notes

1.6. Ask for permission to switch on the recorder

2. Identifying Particulars

2.1. What is your name?

2.2. What gender do you identify with?

2.3. In what year were you born?

2.4. What race group do you identify with?

2.5. What is your home language?

2.6. What faith do you identify with, if any?

2.7. What is your marital status?

2.8. What is your current living situation?

2.8.1. In which area do you live?

2.8.2. Who lives with you?

2.8.3. How many children do you provide care for?

2.8.4. How much space do you each have?

2.9. What is your current employment status?

2.9.1. How much time do you spend at your job? Do you work from or away from home?

2.10. If you wouldn't mind, I'd like to ask you a few brief questions about your total household income?

2.10.1. How many people are reliant on your monthly total household income?

2.10.2. Would you mind telling me which of the following monthly income brackets you would place your household in? [No income; R0 to R1138 x no of people in household; R1138 x no of people in household to R25 600; R25 600 and above]

2.10.2.1. Whose income makes up this amount?

I am going to move on to asking you questions related to ASD and your child's diagnosis. Just a reminder that you and your child's identity will be protected outside of the interview space.

3.   The ASD Epidemic

3.1.   What is your understanding of ASD and what it is?

3.2.   What, in your understanding, are the causes of ASD?

3.3.   In your experience, what do you think other people think the causes of ASD are?

4. The Diagnostic Process

4.1.   Can you tell me a bit about how your child/ren came to receive a diagnosis of living with ASD?

4.1.1.   Can you describe what your child was like before there was any diagnosis or intervention?

4.1.2.   What emotions did you experience before the diagnosis?

4.1.3.   When did your child/ren receive their official diagnosis and by whom?

4.1.4.   How old was/were your child/ren at this time?

4.1.5.   At the time of diagnosis, was there any discussion with your doctor about whether your child had a high functioning or low functioning form of ASD?

4.1.6.   Which medications, if mentioned previously?

4.1.7.   What emotions did you experience during the diagnosis?

4.1.8.   Did you consult anyone other than the person who officially diagnosed your child/ren?

4.1.9.   What were some of the gaps in the service that you received from your doctor during the diagnostic process, whereby your expectations were not met?

4.2.   Can you tell me about what happened after receiving an official diagnosis?

4.2.1.   How did you feel?

4.2.2.   How did you react?

4.2.3.   What actions did you take?

4.3.   How do you feel about your child's diagnosis now?

4.3.1.   To what degree do you feel that you have found acceptance of the diagnosis?

I would like to ask you some questions relating to your experiences of caring for your child/ren, and how you have dealt with some of the challenges that you have faced, if that's okay? I know that it might be difficult to discuss these challenges, and it might feel like you are complaining about your child. At the same time, all parents experience challenges, and there is no judgement for anything that you share with me.

5.   Challenges and Coping Mechanisms

5.1.   What challenges have you experienced with regard to difficult to manage behaviours at home?

5.1.1. With daily routines and care? Discipline? Other children?

5.1.2. How have you coped with these behaviours at home?

5.1.3. Is there anything you would have done differently?

5.2.   What challenges have you experienced with difficult to manage behaviours at school?

5.2.1. Academically? Socially? With the teachers and staff?

5.2.2. Is/are your child/ren in a school that meets their special needs?

5.2.3. What led to, or has prevented, your child/ren from being at a school that meets their special needs?

5.2.4. If your child/ren is at a school that meets their special needs, did you have to do anything to gain acceptance into this form of schooling?

5.2.5. If your child/ren is at a school that meets their special needs, have you considered any alternate forms of schooling apart from the current one? Why or why not?

5.2.6. What are the positive implications of your child/ren's current form of schooling?

5.2.7. What are the negative implications of your child/ren's current form of schooling?

5.2.8. How have you coped with the difficulties related to schooling?

5.2.9. Is there anything you would have done differently?

5.2.10. Are there any gaps in service delivery that you have experienced, in the city in which you live, related to educating your child/ren?

5.3.   What challenges have you experienced with difficult to manage behaviours In public?

5.3.1. Indoors? Outdoors?

5.3.2. How have you coped with difficult behaviours in public?

5.3.3. Is there anything you would have done differently?

5.4.   What challenges have you experienced with regard to how other people have responded to your child?

5.4.1.   With strangers? With friends? With family?

5.4.1.1. How have you responded in return?

5.4.1.2. How have you felt as a result of these interactions?

5.4.1.3. How have you coped with strangers' responses?

5.4.1.4. Is there anything you would have done differently?

5.4.1.5. In your experience, what do you think strangers' understanding is of ASD (behaviours, management, causes)?

5.5.   What emotional impact has caring for a child living with ASD had on you?

5.5.1.   Positive impact?

5.5.2.   Negative impact?

5.5.3.   How have you dealt with the emotional impact?

5.5.4.   What do you do for yourself?

5.5.5.   Is there anything you would have done differently?

5.6.   How has caring for a child living with ASD impacted on you practically?

5.6.1.   How have you coped with this?

5.6.2.   Is there anything you would have done differently?

5.7.   What effect has ASD had on your marriage/previous marriage/romantic relationships?

5.7.1.   How have you coped with this?

5.7.2.   What do you do for yourselves as a couple?

5.7.3.   How has the biological father been involved, if at all?

5.7.4.   What support, if any, have you received from your current partner, or the paternal figure in your child's life if there is one?

5.7.5.   Is there anything you would have done differently?

5.8.   Has there been any impact on your finances in caring for a child living with ASD? If so, what impact has it had?

5.8.1.   Have you had any access to additional financial resources as a result of your child's diagnosis, for example a government grant?

5.8.2.   If there has been an impact on you financially, how have you coped with this?

5.8.3.   Is there anything you would have done differently?

5.9.   Has, or is, your child/ren making use of any intervention strategies to manage their ASD?

5.9.1.   What led to making use of these intervention strategies?

5.9.2.   Are there any intervention strategies that you would like to have access to?

5.9.2.1. What, if anything, has prevented you from having access to these interventions?

5.9.3.   How have you coped with finding appropriate intervention strategies?

5.9.4.   Is there anything you would have done differently?

5.9.5.   What are some of the gaps in service delivery regarding appropriate intervention strategies for your child/ren?

5.10.   What challenges have you experienced with regard to your spirituality, or worldview, if any?

5.10.1. How have you coped with these challenges?

5.10.2. Is there anything you would have done differently?

I would like to ask you a few questions about the support that you feel you have, or haven't received, if that's okay?

6.   Support mechanisms

6.1.   How supported have you felt in caring for your child?

6.1.1.   What support have you received from the government, if any? Education department? Medical health professionals, like doctors, nurses, and psychologists? Family? Friends? Other?

6.1.2.   Have you been a part of any ASD support groups?

6.1.2.1. If so, how did you experience the support from this group?

6.1.2.2. What kind of support did you receive?

6.1.2.3. How did you find out about the group?

6.1.2.4. Are you still part of the group? If not, why?

6.1.2.5. How long have you been a part of the group?

6.1.3.   From all of the potential forms of support that we've spoken about, Is there any support that you would like less or more of?

7.   Future

7.1.   When you think about your child's future, what are the feelings that come up for you?

7.2.	What do you worry about with regard to your child's future?
7.3.	How were your hopes and dreams for your child affected by the diagnosis?
7.4.	Which of these hopes and dreams do you think are more difficult for your child now that they've been diagnosed?
7.5.	Which of your hopes and dreams do you believe have changed in a positive way?
7.6.	What new hopes and dreams do you have for your child since the diagnosis?

**8.	Other**

8.1.	What have you learned?
8.2.	What would you recommend to other parents in terms of coping?
8.3.	Is there anything else that you'd like to share with me that you feel we haven't covered?

**9.	Debrief**

9.1.	We have come to the end of our time together.
9.2.	Do you have any questions/comments for me?
9.3.	Refer them if necessary.

Just a reminder that everything that we've spoken about will be kept private and confidential, and the data will only be used for academic purposes in my Masters' book.

Thank you so much for your time and for being open with me about your experiences.